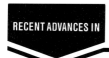

RECENT ADVANCES IN

Obstetrics and Gynaecology

RECENT ADVANCES IN OBSTETRICS AND GYNAECOLOGY

Contents of Number 17
Edited by John Bonnar

ISBN 0443 044023

You can place your order by contacting your local medical bookseller or the Sales Promotion Department, Robert Stevenson House, 1-3 Baxter's Place, Leith Walk, Edinburgh EH1 3AF, UK

Tel: (031) 556 2424; Telex: 727511 LONGMAN G; Fax (031) 558 1278

Look out for *Recent Advances in Obstetrics and Gynaecology 19* in November 1995

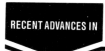

Obstetrics and Gynaecology

Edited by

John Bonnar MA MD (Hons) FRCOG

Professor and Head, Department of Obstetrics and
Gynaecology, University of Dublin; Fellow of Trinity
College, Dublin; Consultant Obstetrician and
Gynaecologist, St James' Hospital
and Coombe Lying-in Hospital, Dublin, Ireland

NUMBER EIGHTEEN

CHURCHILL LIVINGSTONE
EDINBURGH LONDON MADRID MELBOURNE MILAN NEW YORK AND TOKYO 1994

CHURCHILL LIVINGSTONE
Medical Division of Longman Group UK Limited

Distributed in the United States of American by
Churchill Livingstone Inc., 650 Avenue of the Americas, New York,
N.Y. 10011, and by associated companies, branches and
representatives throughout the world.

First published 1994
Reprinted 1994

ISBN 0-443-04870-3
ISSN 0143 6848

British Library Cataloguing in Publication Data
A catalogue record for this book is available from the British Library

Library of Congress Cataloging in Publication Data
is available

Produced by Longman Singapore Publisher Pte Ltd
Printed in Singapore

Contents

Preface

Recent Advances in Obstetrics and Gynaecology aims to provide the practising obstetrician and gynaecologist with an up-to-date review of selected topics with recommendations on clinical management. The contributors to the 18th issue are specialists of international standing who have a major involvement in patient care and in research. This volume contains excellent reviews of many of the most important areas of our specialty. The practising specialist will find a wealth of information with a careful analysis of new knowledge and its significance for improving patient care.

The first section on obstetrics begins with a review of the disease process of pre-eclampsia and current knowledge of the platelet endothelial dysfunction. Dr F. Lyall and Professor I. Greer, Glasgow, provide a detailed appraisal and warn against high expectations of the value of low dose aspirin. The understanding of the antiphospholipid syndrome and its role in recurrent fetal death has been a major advance. For this we owe a great debt to Professor W. Lubbe in Auckland, New Zealand. Dr N. Pattison, Professor W. Lubbe and colleagues examine the new information on antiphospholipid antibodies, their prevalence and role in recurrent fetal death. This group have unique experience in this area and their recommendations for patient management are a welcome advance. We have evolved to a situation where the adverse effects of diabetes in pregnancy are now virtually preventable. Mr. M. Gillmer and Mr N. Bickerton, Oxford, describe how the obstetrician using a team approach can provide the essential supervision of diabetic mothers with the aid of simple technology to give constant patient feedback and strict control of the plasma glucose throughout pregnancy. The diagnosis and management of fetal distress in labour continues as one of the most difficult areas of obstetric practice. Dr G. Mires and Dr N. Patel, Dundee, examine critically the current labour ward practices and the new techniques which are being researched to provide more information on fetal health and metabolism during labour. The obstetric section concludes with an analysis of current litigation for malpractice in our speciality by Dr R. Doherty and Dr C. James of the Medical Defence Union. They explain why many of the claims are not defensible. Many obstetricians and gynaecologists are called upon to provide expert reports in cases of mishap. Sound recommendations are made for such reports. This chapter should be compulsory reading for all who practise in obstetrics and gynaecology.

The second section deals with fertility. Dr G. Baker and Dr E. Keogh, Perth, Australia, provide a comprehensive review of the investigation and management of male infertility. This is often a difficult area for the gynaecologist and clear guidelines are provided for patient management. The distressing subject of recurrent abortion is reviewed by Dr C. Barry-Kinsella and Professor R. Harrison, Dublin. Perhaps they are a little pessimistic about the advances which have been made in this area. In practice, many will agree with their view that where no explanation can be found patients may wish to opt for empirical treatment. The chapter by Ms B. Mostyn, Infertility Counsellor, Guy's Hospital, London, makes salutory reading for all gynaecologists who treat the infertile couple. We are reminded of the distress which can be aggravated by or even caused by the gynaecologist treating the infertile couple. The experiences related by Ms Mostyn emphasize the great need for counselling as an integral part of the management of the infertile couple.

The final section deals with specific areas of gynaecological practice. Teenage women are now seen much more frequently in gynaecological clinics. Miss P. Blomfield, Staffordshire, and Dr I. Duncan, Dundee, examine whether cervical screening is indicated in the sexually active teenager. The evidence provided strongly supports their view that cervical screening is not warranted in this age group. From Manchester, Dr R. Hunter and Dr A. Brewster provide a thorough examination of the advances in diagnostic imaging which enable more effective treatment for advanced carcinoma of the cervix. Ovarian cancer is the most common gynaecological malignancy. The contribution of Dr L. Stewart, Medical Research Council Cancer Trials Office, Cambridge, and Dr. D. Guthrie, Derby, provides an outstanding chapter, analysing the results of chemotherapy for advanced ovarian cancer. Progress in this area is much less than many clinicians appreciate and patient survival is unchanged. I would endorse the recommendation of Drs Stewart and Guthrie that all gynaecologists dealing with ovarian cancer should consider enrolling their patients in the large trials which are at present under way. This scientific approach provides a high standard of treatment and care which can only be of benefit to patients, present and future. It is only by large multi-centre trials that we can hope to lay the foundations for good clinical practice.

The volume concludes with two chapters from individuals with unique experience in their subject. Dr R. Boronow, Jackson, Mississippi, has extensive experience in the management of patients with endometrial cancer. He provides a careful analysis of the evolution of staging of endometrial cancer. Clearly he has serious reservations concerning the current FIGO staging of endometrial cancer. His approach to the staging of the disease and the risk of metastatic spread is entirely logical. The application of this information to the individual patient should determine the extent of both surgery and radiotherapy. A detailed protocol for patient management is provided by Dr Boronow.

The last chapter is by Mr R. Turner-Warwick, London, and Mr C. Chapple, Sheffield. We would all recognize Mr Turner-Warwick as the doyen of uro-gynaecology with a special interest in the management of obstetric and gynaecological injuries to the ureter and the bladder. These complications are a common cause of litigation against gynaecologists. Many of these mishaps are avoidable and their prevention is emphasized. Based on unparalleled experience, the surgical procedures to correct bladder and ureteric fistulas are described. I am most grateful to the authors for this outstanding chapter with its excellent advice for the gynaecologist.

Recent Advances in Obstetrics and Gynaecology 18 has been a pleasure to edit and I hope that you the reader will find it a valuable addition to the series. I wish to thank all the contributors who have provided such a wealth of information. I am indebted to Yvonne O'Leary of Churchill Livingstone for her assistance and for ensuring rapid publication.

Dublin 1994   J. B.

Contributors

H.W. Gordon Baker MB BS PhD FRACP
Senior Research Fellow, Department of Obstetrics and Gynaecology, Royal Women's Hospital, Clayton, Victoria, Australia

Carole Barry-Kinsella MRCPI MRCOG
Lecturer, Royal College of Surgeons in Ireland, Rotunda Hospital, Dublin, Ireland

Nigel J. Bickerton MB BS MRCOG
Formerly Registrar, John Radcliffe Maternity Hospital, Oxford, UK

Mary A. Birdsall MB ChB MRNZCO
Registrar, Department of Obstetrics and Gynaecology, National Women's Hospital, Auckland, New Zealand

P.I. Blomfield MB BS MRCOG
Senior Registrar in Obstetrics and Gynaecology, West Midlands Regional Health Authority, UK

Richard C. Boronow MD
Clinical Professor, Gynaecology, University of Mississippi Medical Center, Jackson, Mississippi, USA

Alison Brewster BSc MD FRCR
Senior Registrar, Department of Radiotherapy, Christie Hospital, Manchester, UK

Lawrence W. Chamley BSc MSc PhD
Research Officer in Reproductive Immunology, Department of Obstetrics and Gynaecology, University of Auckland, Auckland, New Zealand

Christopher R. Chapple BSc MD FRCS FRCS (Urol)
Consultant Reconstructive Urological Surgeon, Royal Hallamshire Hospital, Sheffield, UK

Roger P. Doherty FRCOG FACS
Formerly Secretary for Ireland, Medical Defence Union, London, UK

Ian D. Duncan MB ChB FRCOG
Reader and Honorary Consultant, Department of Obstetrics and
Gynaecology, Ninewells Hospital and Medical School, Dundee, UK

Michael D. G. Gillmer MA MD FRCOG
Honorary Lecturer, Nuffield Department of Obstetrics and
Gynaecology, and Consultant Obstetrician and Gynaecologist,
John Radcliffe Hospital, Oxford, UK

Ian A. Greer MD MRCP (UK) MRCOG
Muirhead Professor and Head, Department of Obstetrics
and Gynaecology, Glasgow Royal Infirmary, Glasgow, UK

David Guthrie PhD FRCOG FRCR
Consultant in Clinical Oncology, Derbyshire Royal Infirmary,
Derby, UK

Robert F. Harrison MD FRCS(Edin) FRCOG FRCPI
Professor and Head, Department of Obstetrics and Gynaecology,
Royal College of Surgeons in Ireland, Rotunda Hospital,
Dublin, Ireland

Robert D. Hunter FRCP (Edin) FRCR
Director of Radiotherapy, Christie Hospital NHS Trust, Withington,
Manchester, UK

Catherine E. James MB ChB FRCOG
Medical Secretariat, Medical Defence Union, London, UK

E. J. Keogh MB BS PhD FRACP
Medical Director, Reproductive Research Institute, and Head,
Department of Endocrinology and Diabetes, Sir Charles Gairdner Hospital,
Nedlands, Western Australia

Wilhelm F. Lubbe MD FCPSA FRACP FACC
Professor of Cardiovascular Studies, Department of Medicine, University of
Auckland, Auckland, New Zealand

Fiona Lyall BSc PhD
Lecturer, Department of Obstetrics and Gynaecology, Royal Infirmary,
Glasgow, UK

Gary J. Mires MB ChB MRCOG
Senior Lecturer, Department of Obstetrics and Gynaecology, University of
Dundee, Dundee, UK

Barbara Mostyn BA MA (Psychol)
Infertility Counsellor, St Thomas's Hospital, London, UK

Naren Patel FRCOG
Honorary Senior Lecturer and Consultant Obstetrician,
Department of Obstetrics and Gynaecology, Ninewells Hospital
and Medical School, Dundee, UK

Neil S. Pattison MD FRNZCOG FRCOG
Senior Lecturer, Department of Obstetrics and Gynaecology,
University of Auckland, Auckland, New Zealand

Lesley A. Stewart BSc MSc PhD
Overview Coordinator, Medical Research Council Cancer Trials Office,
Cambridge, UK

Richard Turner-Warwick CBE DM (Oxon) MCh DSc FRCP FRCS
FRCOG FACS FRACS (Hon)
Emeritus Surgeon, Middlesex Hospital, London; Senior Consultant
Urological Surgeon, St Peter's Group Hospitals, London; Senior Lecturer,
Institute of Urology, London, UK

Obstetrics

1

Is pre-eclampsia a preventable disease?

F. Lyall   I. A. Greer

Pre-eclampsia is a multisystem disorder affecting virtually every organ and system in the body. Hypertension and proteinuria, the traditional diagnostic features, represent only two facets of a complex pathophysiological process. The common pathological feature of the disease, whether in the placental bed, renal microvasculature or cerebral circulation, is vascular endothelial damage and dysfunction. If we wish to prevent such a disorder, then we must seek ways of preventing or ameliorating the disease process. Such a strategy presupposes that we understand the pathophysiological mechanisms underlying the clinical problem. It is believed that endothelial damage and dysfunction may be related to the platelet activation which occurs in pre-eclampsia, and anti-platelet therapy has recently been employed in an attempt to prevent the disorder. This chapter will discuss the pathophysiological processes of pre-eclampsia and the effect of anti-platelet therapy.

COAGULATION CHANGES ASSOCIATED WITH PRE-ECLAMPSIA

Widespread deposition of fibrin associated with vascular damage such as acute atherosis in the placental bed or glomerular endotheliosis has long been known to be a pathological feature of pre-eclampsia, suggesting that the coagulation system is activated (Davies & Prentice 1992, Greer 1992). This is unlikely to be a primary phenomenon, and probably represents a secondary effect consequent to vascular damage. Routine coagulation tests such as the prothrombin time and activated partial thromboplastin time are essentially normal, unless pre-eclampsia is complicated by full-blown disseminated intravascular coagulation (DIC) (Davies & Prentice 1992), as these tests are relatively insensitive to minor changes in coagulation. Elevated levels of fibrinopeptide A (Douglas et al 1982), a sensitive indicator of coagulation activation which is cleaved from fibrinogen by the action of thrombin, suggests that fibrinogen breakdown occurs in severe disease. Fibrinogen itself also increases in hypertensive compared to normal pregnancy (Howie et al 1971), although this may simply be an acute-phase reactant increasing in response to the disease in general. There is an increase in factor VIIIc activity

3

(Howie et al 1971, 1976), but the increase in von Willebrand factor antigen (previously termed factor VIII-related antigen) is greater (Redman et al 1977b). These two substances are distinct entities which join together in the circulation to form a macromolecular complex. Factor VIII is produced by the liver, while von Willebrand's factor is synthesized by the vascular endothelium and increases following endothelial damage. This increase in von Willebrand's factor may therefore reflect endothelial damage.

Activation of the coagulation cascade is usually associated with activation of the fibrinolytic system, and this is true for pre-eclampsia (Davies & Prentice 1992). Concentrations of fibrinogen–fibrin degradation products (Howie et al 1971) and soluble fibrinogen–fibrin complexes (Edgar et al 1977) are increased. The activity of plasminogen activators initially appeared to be normal or slightly reduced in pre-eclampsia compared to normal pregnancy (Howie et al 1971, Bonnar et al 1971), but more precise assays of plasminogen activators and their inhibitors have recently shown unchanged plasma plasminogen activator, but increased levels of tissue plasminogen activator in plasma (Estelles et al 1987). This may be due to stimulation of or damage to the endothelium. This increase in tissue plasminogen activator is accompanied by an increase in plasminogen activator inhibitors 1 and 2 (Estelles et al 1987). Plasminogen activator inhibitor 2 is produced only from the placenta and is not found in plasma from non-pregnant subjects. The increase in this placental plasminogen activator inhibitor may again reflect placental vascular damage and would predispose to local thrombosis by local inhibition of fibrinolysis in the abnormal vessels of the placental bed. Not all studies have been consistent, however; de Boer et al (1988) found an increase in total plasminogen activator inhibitor in pre-eclampsia, with a reduction in the placentally derived inhibitor component compared to normal. They also showed that low levels of placental plasminogen activator inhibitor are associated with poor fetal outcome and might, therefore, simply be a measure of placental function.

The increase in fibrinopeptide β1–42 provides additional evidence of fibrinolytic activation. This peptide is generated by plasmin degradation of fibrin I, a soluble intermediate between fibrinogen and the spontaneously polymerizing fibrin II (Borok et al 1984). Plasminogen (Spencer et al 1983) and the inhibitor of plasmin, α_2-antiplasmin (Oian et al 1985), have also been found to be reduced, in keeping with fibrinolytic activation. This increase in fibrinolysis may be a response to intravascular coagulation which may be prevented from reaching its full potential due to the concomitant increase in intravascular inhibitors of plasminogen activation.

Platelets

Platelets play a crucial role in the pathophysiology of pre-eclampsia by promoting vascular damage and obstruction, leading to tissue ischaemia and further damage (Greer 1992). Thromboxane A_2, the major product of arachidonic acid metabolism in platelets, is a potent vasoconstrictor and platelet-aggregating agent. As it has a short half-life it is normally measured as its stable hydration product, thromboxane B_2. The effects of thromboxane A_2 are normally counterbalanced by prostacyclin, a potent vasodilator and anti-platelet prostanoid which is the major product of arachidonic acid metabolism in vascular endothelium and which plays an important role in protecting the endothelium and limiting damage by inhibiting platelet aggregation and promoting vasodilation. These two substances function as local hormones and are thought to be important in the control of the platelet–endothelium interaction. They oppose each other through the regulation of platelet adenylate cyclase, which controls cAMP production and thereby platelet free calcium concentration; this links receptor occupancy with cellular response. Pro-aggregatory substances such as thromboxane A_2 inhibit adenylate cyclase, allowing free intracellular calcium to rise, while prostacyclin stimulates adenylate cyclase thus increasing cAMP, reducing free intracellular calcium and inhibiting platelet activation.

There is considerable evidence implicating platelets in the pathophysiology of pre-eclampsia. The circulating platelet count is reduced (Redman et al 1978), reflecting a reduced platelet life-span (Rakoczi et al 1979), and an inverse relationship between platelet count and fibrinogen–fibrin degradation products has been noted, suggesting that the reduction in platelet count is due to increased platelet consumption associated with low-grade DIC (Howie et al 1971). The platelet-specific protein β-thromboglobulin, a marker of platelet activation in vivo, has also been found to be increased in pregnancy-induced hypertension (Redman et al 1977a, Douglas et al 1982, Socol et al 1985, Ballegeer et al 1992). This correlates with proteinuria and serum creatinine (Socol et al 1985), and suggests a link between platelet activation with renal microvascular damage.

The platelet content of 5-hydroxytryptamine (5-HT) is reduced in pre-eclampsia, indicating platelet aggregation and stimulation of the platelet release reaction in vivo. Low platelet 5-HT levels have also been associated with loss of platelet responsiveness to various aggregating agents in vitro. The explanation suggested for these findings is that platelets are activated in the micro-circulation of the placenta, kidney and liver, release their products such as β-thromboglobulin and 5-HT, and then re-enter the system in an 'exhausted' state, unable to respond normally to aggregating agents and containing lower levels of 5-HT (Howie 1977). In support of this hypothesis, placentae from patients with pre-eclampsia have been shown to contain high levels of 5-HT, possibly of platelet origin. Other studies using platelet aggregation in platelet-rich plasma have also noted 'platelet exhaustion' (Ahmed et al 1991). This platelet exhaustion phenomenon has also been noted in molar pregnancy complicated by severe hypertension, where anti-platelet therapy corrected the hypofunctional platelet response (Greer et al 1987).

Increased platelet thromboxane A_2 production ex vivo has been shown to occur in pre-eclampsia complicated by intrauterine growth retardation (Wallenburg & Rotmans 1982). More recently, a whole blood platelet aggregation technique has been used to study platelet reactivity (Greer et al 1988). This technique, which leaves platelets in their natural milieu, surrounded by red cells and white cells which may themselves influence the aggregation response, may be a more physiological method than the traditional turbidometric techniques which use platelet-rich plasma. This study showed that platelet reactivity is enhanced in pregnancy-induced hypertension compared to normal pregnant and non-pregnant women. However, Louden et al (1991) found reduced platelet reactivity in whole blood in women with pre-eclampsia compared to normal controls, although there was no difference in thromboxane A_2 production ex vivo. The report of Louden et al (1991) would be in keeping with platelet exhaustion secondary to increased activation in vivo as discussed above, and the differences in results between studies may reflect differences in patient severity, as platelet reactivity may vary according to the stage of the disease process, with increased reactivity perhaps occurring in the early stages of the disease and platelet exhaustion in advanced disease.

The changes in the coagulation system and in platelet function support the concept that disseminated intravascular coagulation occurs in patients with pregnancy-induced hypertension. A 'coagulation index' of serum fibrin–fibrinogen degradation products, platelet count and plasma factor VIII has been shown to correlate with a 'clinical index' of disease severity (Howie et al 1976), highlighting the association of the two conditions.

THE ENDOTHELIUM IN PRE-ECLAMPSIA

The vascular endothelium forms the lining of the circulatory system in all vertebrates and comprises a dynamic unicellular interface between the surrounding vascular cells and the soluble and cellular components of the blood. The vascular endothelium, in response to diverse stimuli, synthesizes and secretes vasoactive agents that influence vascular tone and blood cell interaction. Thus the endothelium is not simply an inert container for circulating blood; it plays an active role in the control of haemostasis and thrombosis and vascular tone (Greer 1992). It produces prostacyclin and endothelium-derived relaxing factor (EDRF), which can inhibit the activation of platelets and neutrophils, and substances such as tissue plasminogen activator which prevent or limit coagulation and vascular damage. Conversely, the endothelium can render itself thrombogenic by secreting von Willebrand's factor, platelet-activating factor and plasminogen activator inhibitor, which promote local coagulation and repair at the site of injury. Vascular tone is under the influence of the endothelium by release of vasodilator substances such as prostacyclin and EDRF and vasoconstrictors such as endothelin. In the normal situation, the endothelium, platelets and neutrophils will interact homeostatically. Although it has long been appreciated that denudation of the endothelium will result in thrombosis, endothelial dysfunction may have similar effects and could transform the endothelium from a non-thrombogenic to a thrombogenic surface. There is now considerable evidence linking endothelial dysfunction to pre-eclampsia (Greer 1992).

Prostacyclin is a potent vasodilator, inhibitor of platelet aggregation and a stimulator of renin secretion. The pathological features of pre-eclampsia are the opposite to these: vasoconstriction, platelet consumption and low renin secretion. In addition, women with pre-eclampsia are very sensitive to exogenous angiotensin II infusions when compared to normal pregnant women (Gant et al 1973); the insensitivity to angiotensin II seen in normal pregnancy can be abolished by treatment with a cyclooxygenase inhibitor such as indomethacin (Everett et al 1978), and enhanced by infusion of prostacyclin (Broughton-Pipkin et al 1984) or prostaglandin E_2 (Broughton Pipkin et al 1982). These experiments suggest that in normal pregnancy angiotensin II may be balanced by the action of vasodepressor prostaglandins such as prostacyclin. A deficiency of prostacyclin might therefore result in the angiotensin II sensitivity seen in pre-eclampsia.

Maternal vascular prostacyclin production is reduced in pre-eclampsia (Bussolino et al 1980), and plasma and urinary prostacyclin metabolites are significantly lower, particularly in those with severe disease (Moodley et al 1984, Goodman et al 1982, Greer 1985, Greer et al 1985). Platelet thromboxane A_2 production may be increased in pre-eclampsia complicated by intrauterine growth retardation (Wallenburg & Rotmans 1982), although Louden et al (1991) found no difference in thromboxane production between normal and hypertensive pregnancies. The resulting imbalance between these two prostanoids, prostacyclin and thromboxane, is likely to contribute to the enhanced platelet reactivity and vascular damage seen in pre-eclampsia.

On the fetal side, production of prostacyclin from cord vessels is reduced in pre-eclampsia (Remuzzi et al 1979, Downing et al 1980, Walsh 1985). Furthermore placentae taken from pregnancies complicated by pre-eclampsia have been shown to produce more thromboxane A_2 and less prostacyclin than those from normal pregnancies (Walsh 1985). Intact umbilical arteries taken from pregnancies complicated by pre-eclampsia have been shown to be unresponsive to a stimulus of prostacyclin production when compared with normal umbilical arteries (McLaren et al 1986, 1987), suggesting that the ability of the vascular endothelium to produce prostacyclin in response to a physiological stimulus is absent or substantially diminished in pre-eclampsia. Since the umbilical artery lacks any innervation it may depend on humoral control of blood flow by prostanoids (Tuvemo 1980) to maintain the low-pressure high-flow feto-placental circulation. Failure of the vessel to produce prostacyclin in response to physiological stimulation may result in increased umbilical artery resistance due to vasoconstriction, especially in the face of increased thromboxane production by the placenta. The deficiency of prostacyclin and resulting prostanoid imbalance may also allow vascular damage to occur unchecked. The mechanism underlying prostacyclin deficiency is unclear, but it may be due to reduced activity of enzyme systems required for its production. These enzymes could be inactivated by free radicals or proteolytic enzymes, making the prostacyclin deficiency a feature of endothelial damage and dysfunction; other markers of endothelial damage, such as elevated levels of fibronectin and laminin (Ballegeer et al 1992), endothelin (Greer et al 1991c, Nova et al 1991) and increased concentrations of von Willebrand's factor and plasminogen activator inhibitors, are also found in pre-eclampsia, emphasizing the extent of the endothelium damage and dysfunction which occurs in this disorder.

In 1980 a labile endothelium-derived compound was discovered to play an important role as part of a signal transduction pathway linking agents acting on the endothelium with relaxation of the underlying smooth muscle (Furchgott & Zawadzki 1980) and was termed EDRF. EDRF was subsequently shown to be the inorganic free radical gas nitric oxide (NO) (Palmer et al 1987). It is the most potent known vasodilator identified to date and its synthesis has been discovered in a striking diversity of tissues and cultured cells (Moncada et al 1991). EDRF is derived from L-arginine by the action of NO synthase. In all enzyme isoforms so far identified it involves oxidation of one of the terminal guanidino nitrogens of L-arginine to yield NO plus L-citrulline (Marletta 1989). There are at least two types of NO synthase (Moncada et al 1991). In many tissues, including vascular endothelium and brain, basal NO synthetic activity rapidly increases in response to activation of specific cell surface receptors. These constitutive NO synthases are stimulated by calcium/calmodulin, and the rapid increase in enzyme activity is not dependent on new protein synthesis. By contrast, activation of NO synthase in macrophages and leucocytes and also in endothelium occurs over several hours in response to specific cytokines. These inducible NO synthases are calcium/calmodulin independent and require new protein synthesis.

The physiological role of EDRF synthesis in the control of blood flow and blood pressure in man has been demonstrated by use of inhibitors of NO synthase (Moncada et al 1991, Vallance et al 1989).

Adaptation of the maternal cardiovascular system to pregnancy is characterized by a reduction in peripheral vascular resistance and a fall in blood pressure, the latter reaching a nadir at 20 weeks gestation and increasing towards non-pregnant levels in the third trimester. Pre-eclampsia occurs in around 5% of pregnancies. Although NO plays an important role in the control of systemic blood pressure, the role of NO in human pregnancy has not been widely assessed. It was recently demonstrated that the perfused human placenta is capable of both generating and responding to NO (Myatt et al 1991). In addition inhibition of NO generation increased perfusion pressure of the feto-placental circulation, suggesting basal release of NO contributes to vascular tone in the placental villus vascular tree. A calcium/ calmodulin-dependent endothelial isoform of NO synthase has recently been characterized in the human villous vascular tree (Myatt et al 1992). In perfused umbilical vessels taken from women with pregnancy-induced hypertension, release of EDRF in response to bradykinin was reduced (Pinto et al 1991). NO is an inhibitor of platelet activation (Moncada et al 1991), and impairment of its formation in the vessel wall will not only predispose to vasoconstriction but will also favour platelet adhesion, aggregation and the consequent release of vasoconstrictor substances.

NO synthesis can be determined by measuring urinary levels of nitrites and nitrates — oxidation products of NO. Increases in levels of urinary nitrites and nitrates have been demonstrated during elevation of blood pressure in rats (Suzuki et al 1992). Recently the oxidation products of NO — nitrites and nitrates — have been measured in the urine of normal pregnant and hypertensive pregnant women (Cameron et al 1993). No difference in nitrite and nitrate levels was found between the hypertensive and normotensive women; however, in the hypertensive women there was a direct correlation between urinary nitrite/nitrate excretion and the change in systolic blood pressure, suggesting a compensatory increase in NO synthesis in pregnant women to maintain homeostasis.

Hypoxia inhibits NO release from vascular rings (Muramatsu et al 1992). Thus it is possible that ischaemia-induced inhibition of EDRF is responsible for some aspects of the increased placental vascular resistance observed in pre-eclampsia. Although it is clear that NO plays a role in the placenta, it is not yet clear that it has a causative role in placental pathologies. Further studies are thus required.

NEUTROPHIL ACTIVATION

Neutrophils are involved in the pathophysiology of vascular damage in non-pregnant individuals. Activated neutrophils release a variety of substances capable of mediating vascular damage, including the contents of neutrophil granules such as elastase and other proteases. These can destroy the integrity of the endothelial cells, vascular basement membrane and subendothelial matrix (Harlan 1987). Toxic oxygen species are also released, and can produce membrane lipid perodixation, lysis of endothelial cells, and increased vascular permeability and reactivity (Harlan 1987). Leukotrienes are also synthesized and released following neutrophil activation and they too will increase vascular permeability, induce vasoconstriction, and promote further neutrophil activation and adherence (Bray 1983).

Neutrophil elastase, a marker of neutrophil activation in vivo, is elevated in pre-eclampsia, indicating the presence of neutrophil activation (Greer et al 1989a), but this is confined to the maternal circulation (Greer et al 1991b). As elevated neutrophil elastase is found in both mild/moderate and severe disease it may be an early feature of the disease process (Greer et al 1989a). The elevated levels of neutrophil elastase seen in pre-eclampsia correlate with the increase in plasma von Willebrand factor and are associated with an increase in the endothelial-derived vasoconstrictor endothelin (Greer et al 1991c). Neutrophil activation may therefore contribute directly to the vascular lesions seen in pre-eclampsia, such as those noted in the placental bed. Elastase-positive neutrophils can be found in significantly increased numbers in the decidua of the placental bed in women with pre-eclampsia compared to normal pregnancies and this correlates with plasma urate, an established marker of disease activity (Butterworth et al 1991). In addition to directly bringing about endothelial damage, neutrophils will interact with platelet, coagulation and complement systems. The activation of neutrophils in pre-eclampsia is likely to be a secondary phenomenon, possibly triggered by the immunological mechanisms which have been implicated in the aetiology of this disorder, or simply secondary to vascular damage and endothelial dysfunction per se; nonetheless it may be an important contributor to the pathogenesis of this disease.

It is of interest that neutrophil granule enzymes (Miller et al 1985), reactive oxygen species (Ager & Gordon 1984) and leukotrienes (Pologe et al 1984) have been shown to stimulate prostacyclin release from endothelial cells. This seems paradoxical since pre-eclampsia is associated with a deficiency of prostacyclin production, which is thought to contribute to the platelet consumption and vasoconstriction seen in the condition. It is known that low concentrations of reactive oxygen species can stimulate cyclooxygenase, which is essential for prostacyclin production, but higher concentrations will inhibit both this enzyme and prostacyclin synthase (Warso & Lands 1983). Furthermore high concentrations of reactive oxygen species can reorientate the arachidonic acid pathway in the cell away from the production of the cytoprotective and vasodilator agent prostacyclin towards thromboxane A_2 (Warso & Lands 1983). Thus neutrophil activation may account for the necrotizing arteriopathy of pre-eclampsia which has hitherto been poorly explained, and may also explain several other features of the disease, such as prostacyclin deficiency and enhanced thromboxane production. Such neutrophil activation is not specific to pre-eclampsia, as increased neutrophil elastase has been found in diabetic pregnancy (Greer et al 1989b) and in mothers with pregnancies complicated by intrauterine growth retardation (Johnston et al 1991).

It has been noted that serum from women with pre-eclampsia has a greater mitogenic effect on fibroblast cells (Roberts et al 1991) and a greater cytotoxic effect on cultured endothelial cells than serum from normal pregnancies (Rodgers et al 1988). Although the nature of this factor is unclear, the authors suggest that, as this effect diminishes following delivery, it may be released from the placenta, but it could equally well be related to neutrophil activation. Furthermore, incubation of monolayer cultures of human umbilical vein endothelial cells with sera from pre-eclamptic women caused significantly greater increases in cellular fibronectin, an important mediator of platelet adhesion and aggregation, than post-delivery pre-eclamptic sera or pre-delivery or post-delivery normal pregnancy sera. No effect was observed on tissue factor, a procoagulant protein, or on von Willebrand factor, known to be deposited in areas of endothelial injury, where it mediates platelet adhesion at these sites (Taylor et al 1991). Thus sera from pre-eclamptic women appeared to induce a selective activation of endothelial cell procoagulant protein production in vitro. Evidence that poor placental perfusion results in production of factor(s) by the placenta which activates/injuries endothelial cells has been reviewed elsewhere (Friedman et al 1991, Roberts et al 1991). It has been reported that human pregnancy serum causes a higher rate of decidual endothelial cell replication when compared to control serum (Gallery et al 1991). However, in these experiments the control serum used was obtained from fetal calf rather than human. Comparison between normal and hypertensive serum on these cells has not yet been performed. There is also evidence of a serum factor in pre-eclampsia which can increase vascular reactivity to angiotensin II in vitro (Tulenko et al 1987).

From the foregoing discussion, it is clear that endothelial damage and dysfunction are common features of all of the pathological features of pre-eclampsia whether in the uteroplacental bed or in the renal microcirculation. The biochemical evidence of endothelial damage includes elevated von Willebrand factor and fibronectin levels, which are released when endothelial cell injury occurs, and reduced prostacyclin production. Functionally, the vessels have an exaggerated response to angiotensin II and there is increased capillary permeability. Endothelial damage and dysfunction stimulate activation of platelets and the coagulation system, promoting further vascular damage. Neutrophils can also be activated by dysfunctional endothelium. Activation of platelets and the coagulation system can cause endothelial damage directly, and also indirectly by activation of neutrophils. If neutrophils are activated they will produce endothelial damage directly, and also indirectly, by platelet activation. Thus endothelial damage, the platelets and coagulation system, and neutrophils all interact; once one of these systems is triggered a positive feedback loop will promote vascular damage. The trigger which initiates this vicious circle is unclear. It appears to originate in the placenta or uteroplacental bed and is probably linked to the failure of trophoblast invasion which is characteristic of the disease (Pijnenborg et al 1991). This process leads to tissue ischaemia, which in turn activates the vicious circle described above to produce widespread endothelial damage and dysfunction. Also obscure is which facet of the vicious circle—endothelial damage, neutrophil activation or platelet activation—is triggered first.

ANTI-PLATELET THERAPY IN THE PREVENTION OF PRE-ECLAMPSIA

The above discussion highlights the complex nature of the disease process of pre-eclampsia. While platelets appear to play a significant role in this process, the disorder can in no way be regarded as simply due to increased platelet reactivity. However, anti-platelet therapy may still influence the disease process by interrupting the vicious cycle described above. Aspirin is the most practicable and effective agent presently available for clinical use as anti-platelet therapy. Small-scale studies suggest that it may be effective in the prevention of pre-eclampsia and intrauterine growth retardation. The biggest problem with regard to its use is perhaps that of identifying patients who will require such therapy; this is especially true in pre-eclampsia, where those with the most severe disease are often primigravidae.

Aspirin acts by irreversibly inhibiting cyclooxygenase, which is required for prostaglandin and thromboxane production, and reducing thromboxane generation and platelet activation. However, the beneficial effects of aspirin may be offset by its inhibition of vascular prostacyclin production, as cyclooxygenase is required for the production of both substances (Greer et al 1986). This is clearly undesirable in pre-eclampsia. However, low-dose aspirin may selectively block thromboxane production. Aspirin is extensively metab-olized by the liver, and low doses given orally are thought to produce pharmacologically active drug concentrations in the portal circulation and not in the systemic circulation. Since platelet cyclooxygenase is irreversibly inhibited by aspirin, effective inhibition of platelet function would result as the platelet passes through the portal circulation, while systemic vascular prostacyclin production might remain unaffected due to lower concentrations in the systemic circulation. In addition the nucleated vascular endothelial cells, unlike anucleate platelets, can synthesize new protein and are therefore able to replace any inactivated enzyme in a matter of hours (Heavey et al 1985), thus maintaining prostacyclin production.

The efficacy of low-dose aspirin in reducing thromboxane A_2 production has largely been demonstrated in non-pregnant patients; doses as low as 20 mg per day reduce thromboxane A_2 production by up to 95% (Sinzinger et al 1989). However, it seems unlikely that any dose of aspirin can produce maximal inhibition of platelet thromboxane A_2 production without affecting prostacyclin production to some extent, although there appears to be a high degree of relative sparing of prostacyclin production with low-dose aspirin (Fitzgerald et al 1983, 1987).

Perhaps the biggest concern regarding the use of aspirin in pregnancy is that of aspirin reaching the fetus and impairing haemostasis or closing the ductus arteriosus, especially near to the time of delivery. The transfer of aspirin has been examined in the perfused human placental cotyledon (Jacobson et al 1991). Aspirin (10^{-5} mol/l) was transferred rapidly from maternal to fetal circuits, but had no effect on resting perfusion pressure of either maternal or fetal circulation. Stuart et al (1982) have documented haemostatic problems in neonates whose mothers received large doses (5–10 g) of aspirin up to 5 days before delivery. Ritter et al (1987) found that 37.5 mg aspirin administered daily for 2 weeks prior to the expected date of delivery significantly lowered maternal thromboxane A_2 but had no signifi-cant effect on thromboxane A_2 in neonatal blood or on prostacyclin production by the umbilical artery ex vivo. This differential effect is likely to reflect the extensive first-pass metabolism of aspirin in the liver, although significant levels of active aspirin can be detected in maternal plasma 1 hour after doses as low as 37.5 and 75 mg (Greer et al 1991a). Chronic maternal intake of 60 mg aspirin daily was also shown to have no significant effect on neonatal platelet function (Louden et al 1989). Sibai et al (1989) have also shown that chronic maternal therapy with aspirin (20–80 mg per day) has no effect on neonatal platelet function or on the ductus arteriosus. Thus it would appear that low-dose aspirin has a selective effect on maternal platelet function, sparing fetal platelet function and prostacyclin production. It is also reassuring that there is no obvious effect on the ductus arteriosus.

Identification of patients at high risk, especially primigravidae, is a major problem. The possibility that platelet angiotensin II receptors may identify high-risk women (Baker et al 1989, 1991) is an interesting development, as such a simple test could be widely employed, and a positive result used as an indication for low-dose aspirin therapy.

There have now been several studies examining the clinical efficacy of low-dose aspirin in the prevention of pre-eclampsia. The first was that of Beaufils et al (1985), who randomized 102 women at high risk of pre-eclampsia to receive either no therapy or aspirin 150 mg in combination with dipyridamole 300 mg daily. The patients were selected on the basis of their past medical and obstetric histories, such as essential hypertension or a series of complicated pregnancies, and 99 of the women were parous. Spontaneous abortions and loss of patients to follow-up left 93 patients for inclusion in the analysis. There was a significant reduction in pre-eclampsia and an improved perinatal outcome in the treated group; 6 of 45 patients in the control group compared to none of the 48 patients in the treatment group developed pre-eclampsia. The incidence of growth retardation and fetal/neonatal loss was also significantly reduced and there was a significant prolongation of pregnancy. No side-effects except headache associated with dipyridamole therapy, and no haemorrhagic complications were encountered. This study, however, used relatively small numbers of patients and the groups were unbalanced with regard to several variables of prognostic significance, which could bring the results into question. In addition two drugs — aspirin and dipyridamole — were tested in combination, although there is no evidence to suggest that dipyridamole will enhance the clinical effect of aspirin alone. Finally 150 mg per day of aspirin was used; this is substantially more than required to produce effective inhibition of platelet thromboxane A_2 production.

Wallenburg et al (1986) reported their findings on low-dose (60 mg per day) aspirin therapy in women at risk of pre-eclampsia. Patients were selected for inclusion in the double-blind, placebo-controlled trial by screening 207 women with angiotensin II infusions. The 46 who were sensitive to angiotensin II at 28 weeks gestation were recruited to the study; 44 were included in the analysis. While there was a significant reduction in the development of hypertensive complications (2 of 21 in the treatment group versus 12 of 23 in the placebo group) there was no significant effect on length of gestation at delivery or number of growth-retarded infants, although there was a tendency to a lower incidence of these conditions in the treatment group.

Wallenburg et al (1991) hypothesized that if enhanced angiotensin II sensitivity was a pathophysiological factor in the development of pregnancy-induced hypertension caused by prostacyclin–thromboxane A_2 imbalance, then low-dose aspirin might restore refractoriness to angiotensin II in angiotensin II pregnant women. To investigate this a randomized, placebo-controlled, double-blind trial was carried out to elucidate whether low-dose aspirin (60 mg per day), taken from 28–34 weeks gestation would reduce the vasopresssor response to intravenously infused angiotensin II in normotensive, angiotensin-sensitive primigravid women (Wallenburg et al 1991). The 36 patients in the study, who were sensitive to angiotensin II, were selected by screening 142 women with angiotensin infusions. Angiotensin II sensitivity was determined again at 34 weeks gestation. The test was not repeated on 3 women in the placebo group because they became hypertensive before 34 weeks gestation. In the aspirin group all women were normotensive at 34 weeks gestation. In the group taking aspirin, vascular refractoriness to angiotensin II was restored in 14 of the 17 women compared with 5 of the 15 women in the placebo group. The authors proposed that prostacyclin–thromboxane imbalance is important in the development of the enhanced angiotensin sensitivity associated with pregnancy-induced hypertension.

Schiff et al (1989) selected patients on the basis of the 'roll-over test' (Gant et al 1974), although the predictive value of this test is disputed (Phelen et al 1977). After blood pressure has been measured in the left lateral position, the patient rolls on to her back, and after a few minutes the blood pressure measurement is repeated. An increase in diastolic blood pressure of more than 15 mmHg after 'rolling over' is considered positive. After screening 791 women, 65 with positive tests were randomized to receive aspirin 100 mg per day or placebo in a prospective double-blind manner. The patients were of mixed parity. There was a significant reduction in hypertensive complications, an increase in gestation at delivery, and an increase in adjusted birthweight centile compared with the placebo group. There were no maternal side-effects and no maternal or neonatal haemorrhagic effects.

In a further study Schiff et al (1990) performed a prospective, placebo-controlled, randomized double-blind trial of the influence of low-dose aspirin (100 mg per day) treatment in women with mild pregnancy-induced hypertension during the third trimester of pregnancy. From 192 pregnant women suffering from pregnancy-induced hypertension, they selected 47 women with a systolic blood pressure above 140 but below 165 mmHg and/or diastolic blood pressure above 90 but below 110 mmHg, who were nulliparous, had a gestational age of between 30 and 36 weeks and showed no signs of moderate to severe pregnancy-induced hypertension such as a low platelet count (less than 10^5 ml) or proteinuria (>500 mg per day). Women with known sensitivity to aspirin, chronic hypertension, chronic renal disorder or who were on antihypertensive treatment before admission were excluded from the study. About 25% of the women in each group subsequently developed moderate to severe pre-eclampsia. There was no significant differences between the groups with regard to abdominal deliveries, newborn weight or the mean 5-minute Apgar score. The authors concluded that in order to prevent pre-eclampsia preventive treatment should start weeks before clinical signs appear.

Benigni et al (1989) studied the effects of 60 mg aspirin or placebo in 33 women judged to be at risk of pre-eclampsia on the basis of their past obstetric history or past medical history such as chronic hypertension. Treatment was started from the 12th week single-blind. The infants of the treatment group had a significantly greater birthweight and longer gestation than those of the placebo group, but no other differences were noted. Aspirin also significantly and substantially reduced urinary thromboxane B_2 levels, but there was no effect on prostacyclin production, measured as its metabolites in urine, indicating that a selective effect on platelets was occurring, with sparing of the endothelium. Again, no haemorrhagic complications were found in the newborn infants, although there was a significant reduction in serum thromboxane B_2 in the neonates in the treatment group, but this was not as great as the reduction which occurred in the mothers. However, this suggests that even with a dose as low as 60 mg aspirin per day the fetus is still exposed to some active aspirin.

The potential efficacy of anti-platelet therapy with low-dose aspirin is not limited to pre-eclampsia. Pregnancies at risk of intrauterine growth retardation also appear to benefit from such therapy (Wallenburg & Rotmans 1987, Trudinger et al 1988, Uzan et al 1991), as do pregnancies at risk of intrauterine growth retardation and fetal loss because of maternal systemic lupus erythematosus (Elder et al 1988). This is not surprising; all of these disorders are associated with vascular damage in the placental bed.

Recently the effects of low-dose aspirin (100 mg per day) were tested on women with both an abnormal umbilical artery systolic/diastolic ratio on Doppler ultrasound examination and a positive pressor response to angiotensin II (Cook & Trudinger 1993). Of 633 women with an at-risk fetus, 41 were selected based on an abnormal umbilical artery Doppler study result. Of these 41 women, 25 demonstrated a positive pressor response to angiotensin II infusion and were treated with aspirin for the remainder of the pregnancy. The angiotensin II pressor response test was repeated after a minimum of 1 week of treatment. The initial systolic/diastolic ratio was classed as extreme in 8 women and these women retained a positive pressor response to angiotensin II infusion. In the remaining 17 women the initial systolic/diastolic ratio was classed as high. Of these women, 7 converted to a negative pressor response to angiotensin II infusion and exhibited a decreased systolic/diastolic ratio. These women had larger babies and placentae compared with the women who retained a positive pressor response to angiotensin II infusion after aspirin treatment. Larger, placebo-controlled studies will be required to substantiate these findings.

One of the problems of the studies on aspirin prophylaxis for pre-eclampsia is that no study has been large enough to provide the power to assess accurately the benefit (and risks) of aspirin therapy on endpoints such as perinatal mortality. The CLASP study (Collaborative Low-dose Aspirin Study in Pregnancy) was established to assess the effects of anti-platelet administration during pregnancy on substantive measures of maternal and fetal morbidity and perinatal mortality, and this study is due to be completed in the near future. Until such conclusive data are available on the risks and benefits of aspirin use in this situation, we must remain cautious with regard to whether aspirin can prevent pre-eclampsia without risk to mother or fetus. This is emphasized by the findings from a large North American study (Sibai et al 1993). In a recently completed double-blind, placebo-controlled study 3135 healthy pregnant women were randomly assigned at 13–27 weeks gestation to receive 60 mg aspirin per day or a matching placebo. Of these, 150 women (4.8%) were lost to follow-up. The incidence of pre-eclampsia defined as blood pressure of $\geqslant 140$ mmHg systolic and/or 90 mmHg diastolic plus proteinuria ($\geqslant 300$ mg per 24 hours or $\geqslant 2+$ by dipstick, was 26% lower in the aspirin group but this did not reach statistical significance. However, the incidence of abruptio placentae was significantly higher in the aspirin group. There was no difference in birthweight, Caesarean section rate or perinatal death. It was concluded that, because of the increased risk of abruptio placentae, routine use of low-dose aspirin therapy in healthy nulliparous women is unwarranted. Furthermore, the Italian collaborative study (Italian Study of Aspirin in Pregnancy 1993), which recruited over a thousand women at risk of pre-eclampsia and randomized them to receive either 50 mg aspirin daily until delivery or no treatment, found no difference in any of the outcomes measured. These included mean birthweight, birthweight less than the 10th centile for gestation, perinatal mortality, gestation at birth and the development of pregnancy-induced hypertension (PIH) and proteinuria. In addition there was no excesss risk of abruption.

One potential 'surrogate' technique in the absence of such data is to employ meta-analysis of the available studies. Collins (1990) performed such an analysis by conflating the data on all properly randomized trials of anti-platelet therapy in pregnancy. Trials using methods of allocation that did not preclude foreknowledge of trial treatment, e.g. odd/even date of birth or trials with no clinical outcome yet reported, were excluded from the study. The number of participants in these trials was small and the data on the endpoints considered were not yet available from all the studies. There is also concern with regard to reporting bias as studies with a positive outcome are likely to be more readily and rapidly reported than those which are negative, so biasing the assessment of aspirin use in pregnancy. Table 1.1 summarizes the meta-analysis of these studies as reported by Collins (1990). The conclusion of this overview was that, although the results are promising, they must be regarded

Table 1.1 Effect of anti-platelet agents for prevention of intrauterine growth retardation (IUGR) and pre-eclampsia (Reproduced from Collins 1990)

Parameter	No. of trials	Typical odds ratio	95% confidence interval
Hypertension	6	0.57	0.36–0.92
Proteinuric pre-eclampsia	9	0.2	0.11–0.36
Perinatal death	10	0.52	0.21–1.24
Preterm delivery	2	0.22	0.06–0.78
IUGR[a]	6	0.61	0.33–1.15
Caesarean section	5	0.44	0.25–0.76
Intraventricular haemorrhage	9	0.5	0.08–3.11

[a] Birthweight < 5th or 10th centile for gestation.

as far from conclusive. As for implications for current practice, until larger studies such as CLASP have been completed it remains unclear whether or not anti-platelet administration should be adopted in routine clinical practice. The problem of whether or not to use aspirin is worsened by the difficulty in identifying primigravidae at risk of the disorder. Until effective objective techniques for identification of patients at risk are available, the obstetrician must weigh up the available evidence for aspirin's benefits (and potential hazards) against the patient's risk of significant clinical problems and treat the patient as he or she feels appropriate. Therefore the answer to the question of whether pre-eclampsia is a preventable disease is that the case is at present unproven.

REFERENCES

Ager A, Gordon J L 1984 Differential effects of hydrogen peroxide on indices of endothelial cell function. J Exp Med 159: 592–603.

Ahmed Y, Sullivan M H F, Elder M G 1991 Detection of platelet desensitization in pregnancy-induced hypertension is dependent on the agonist used. Thromb Haemost 65: 474–477

Baker P N, Broughton Pipkin F, Symonds E M 1989 Platelet angiotensin II binding sites in hypertension in pregnancy. Lancet ii: 1151 (letter)

Baker P N, Broughton-Pipkin F, Symonds E M 1991 Platelet angiotension II binding sites in normotensive and hypertensive women. Br J Obstet Gynaecol 98: 436–440

Ballegeer V C, Spitz B, De Baene L A et al 1992 Platelet activation and vascular damage in gestational hypertension. Am J Obstet Gynecol 166: 629–633

Beaufils M, Uzan S, Donsimoni R, Colau J C 1985 Prevention of pre-eclampsia by early anti-platelet therapy. Lancet i: 840–842

Benigni A, Gregorini G, Frusca T et al 1989 Effect of low dose aspirin on fetal and maternal generation of thromboxane by platelets in women at risk for pregnancy induced hypertension. N Engl J Med 321: 357–362

Bonnar J, McNicol G P, Douglas A S 1971 Coagulation and fibrinolytic systems in pre-eclampsia. Br Med J 2: 12–16

Borok Z, Weitz J, Owen M et al 1984 Fibrinogen proteolysis and platelet-granule release in pre-eclampsia/eclampsia. Blood 63: 525–531

Bray M A 1983 The pharmacology and pathophysiology of leukotriene B4. Br Med Bull 39: 249–254

Broughton-Pipkin F, Hunter J C, Turner S R et al 1982 Prostaglandin E_2 attenuates the pressor response to angiotensin II in pregnant, but not non-pregnant humans. Am Obstet

Gynecol 142: 168

Broughton-Pipkin F, Morrison R, O'Brien P M S 1984 Effects of prostacyclin on the pressor response to angiotensin II in human pregnancy. Eur J Clin Invest 14: 3

Bussolino F, Benedetto C, Massobrio M, Comussi G 1980 Maternal vascular prostacyclin activity in pre-eclampsia. Lancet ii: 702 (letter)

Butterworth B, Greer I A, Liston W D et al 1991 Immunocytochemical localization of neutrophil elastase in term placenta decidua and myometrium in pregnancy-induced hypertension. Br J Obstet Gynaecol 98: 929–933

Cameron I T, van Papendorp C L, Palmer R M J et al 1993 Relationship between nitric oxide synthesis and increase in systolic blood pressure in women with hypertens in pregnancy. Hypertens Pregnancy 12: 91–98

Collins R 1990 Antiplatelet agents for IUGR and pre-eclampsia. In: Chalmers I (ed) Oxford database of perinatal trials. Version 1.2. disk Issue 4. August 1990. Record 4000

Cook C-M, Trudinger B J 1993 Angiotensin sensitivity predicts aspirin benefit in placental insufficiency. Br J Obstet Gynaecol 100: 46–50

Davies J A, Prentice C R M 1992 Coagulation changes in pregnancy-induced hypertension and growth retardation. In: Greer I A, Turpie A G G, Forbes C D (eds) Haemostasis and thrombosis in obstetrics and gynaecology. Chapman & Hall, London, pp 143–162

de Boer K, Lecander I, ten Cate J W, Borm J J J, Treffers P E 1988 Placental type plasminogen activator inhibitor in pre-eclampsia. Am Obstet Gynecol 158: 518–522

Douglas J T, Shah M, Lowe G D O et al 1982 Plasma fibrinopeptide A and betathromboglobulin in pre-eclampsia and pregnancy hypertension. Thromb Haemost 47: 54–55

Downing I, Shepherd G L, Lewis P J 1980 Reduced prostacyclin production in pre-eclampsia. Lancet ii: 1374 (letter)

Edgar W, McKillop C, Howie P W et al 1977 Composition of soluble fibrin complexes in pre-eclampsia. Thromb Res 10: 567–574

Elder M G, de Swiet M, Robertson A et al 1988 Low dose aspirin in pregnancy. Lancet i: 410 (letter)

Estelles A, Gilabert J, Espana F et al 1987 Fibrinolysis in pre-eclampsia. Fibrinolysis 1: 209–214

Everett R B, Worley R J, MacDonald P C et al 1978 Oral administration of theophylline to modify pressor responsiveness to angiotensin II in women with pregnancy-induced hypertension. Am J Obstet Gynecol 132: 359–362

Fitzgerald G A, Oates J A, Hawiger J et al 1983 Endogenous biosynthesis of prostacyclin and thromboxane and platelet function during chronic administration of aspirin in man. J Clin Invest 71: 676–688

Fitzgerald D J, Mayo G, Catella F et al 1987 Increased thromboxane biosynthesis in normal pregnancy is mainly derived from platelets. Am J Obstet Gynecol 159: 325–330

Friedman S A, Taylor R N, Roberts J M 1991 Pathophysiology of pre-eclampsia. Hypertens Pregnancy 18: 661–682

Furchgott R F, Zawadzki J V 1980 The obligatory role of endothelial cells in the relaxation of arterial smooth muscle by acetycholine. Nature 288: 373–376

Gallery E D M, Rowe J, Schrieber L et al 1991 Isolation and purification of microvascular endothelium from human decidual tissue in the late phase of pregnancy. Am J Obstet Gynecol 165: 191–196

Gant N F, Daley G L, Chand S et al 1973 A study of angiotensin II pressor response throughout primigravid pregnancy. J Clin Invest 52: 2682–2689

Gant N F, Chand S, Worley R J et al 1974 A clinical test useful for predicting the development of acute hypertension in pregnancy. Am J Obstet Gynecol 120: 1–7

Goodman R P, Killam A P, Brash A R et al 1982 Prostacyclin production during pregnancy: comparison of production during normal pregnancy and pregnancy complicated by hypertension. Am J Obstet Gynecol 142: 817–822

Greer I A 1985 The effect of anti-hypertensive agents on platelets, prostacyclin and thromboxane and observations on prostacyclin and thromboxane in normal and hypertensive pregnancy. MD thesis, University of Glasgow

Greer I A 1992 Pathological processes in pregnancy-induced hypertension and intrauterine growth retardation: 'an excess of heated bood'. In Greer I A, Turpie A G G, Forbes C D, (eds) Haemostasis and thrombosis in obstetrics and gynaecology. Chapman & Hall, London, pp 163–202

Greer I A, Walker J J, Cameron A D et al 1985 A prospective longitudinal study of immunoreactive prostacyclin and thromboxane metabolites in normal and hypertensive pregnancies. Clin Exp Hypertens B4: 167–182

Greer I A, Walker J J, Forbes C D et al 1986 The low dose aspirin controversy solved at last? Br Med J 391: 1277–1278

Greer I A, Walker J J, Forbes C D et al 1987 Platelet function in pregnancy induced hypertension following treatment with labetalol and low dose aspirin. Thromb Res 46: 667–612

Greer I A, Calder A A, Walker J J et al 1988 Increased platelet reactivity in pregnancy-induced hypertension and uncomplicated diabetic pregnancy: an indication for anteplatelet therapy? Br J Obstet Gynaecol 95: 1204–1208

Greer I A, Haddad N G, Dawes J, Johnstone F D, Calder A A 1989a Neutrophil activation in pregnancy induced hypertension. Br J Obstet Gynaecol 96: 978–982

Greer I A, Haddad N G, Dawes J et al 1989b Increased neutrophil activation in diabetic pregnancy and non-pregnant diabetic women. Obstet Gynecol 74: 878–881

Greer I A, Gibson J, Brennand J et al 1991a Does low dose aspirin provide a totally selective effect in pregnancy? Br J Haematol 77 (Suppl 1): 5.

Greer I A, Dawes J, Johnston T A et al 1991b Neutrophil activation is confined to the maternal circulation in pregnancy induced hypertension. Obstet Gynecol 78: 28–32

Greer I A, Leask R, Hodson B A et al 1991c Endothelin, elastase and endothelial dysfunction in pre-eclampsia. Lancet i: 558.

Harlan J D 1987 Neutrophil-mediated vascular injury. Acta Med Scand (Suppl) 715: 123–129

Heavey D J, Barrow S E, Hickling N E et al 1985 Aspirin causes short-lived inhibition of bradykinin-stimulated prostacyclin production in man. Nature 318: 186–188

Howie P W 1977 The haemostatic mechanisms of pre-eclampsia. Clin Obstet Gynaecol 4: 595–609

Howie P W, Prentice C R M, McNicol G P 1971 Coagulation, fibrinolysis and platelet function in pre-eclampsia, essential hypertension and placental insufficiency. J Obstet Gynaecol Br Commonw 78: 992–1003

Howie P W, Begg C B, Purdie D W et al 1976 Use of coagulation tests to predict the clinical progress of pre-eclampsia. Lancet ii: 323–325

Italian Study of Aspirin in Pregnancy 1993 Low dose aspirin in prevention and treatment of intrauterine growth retardation and pregnancy-induced hypertension. Lancet 341: 396–400

Jacobson R L, Brewer A, Eis A et al 1991 Transfer of aspirin across the perfused human placental cotyledon. Am J Obstet Gynecol 165: 939–944

Johnston J, Greer I A, Dawes J et al 1991 Neutrophil activation in small for gestational age pregnancies. Br J Obstet Gynaecol 98: 104–105

Louden K A, Heptinstall S, Broughton-Pipkin F et al 1989 The effect of low dose aspirin on platelet reactivity on pregnancy, PIH and neonates. Clin Exp Hypertens B8: 398

Louden K A, Broughton-Pipkin F, Heptinstall S et al 1991 Platelet reactivity and serum thromboxane B_2 production in whole blood in gestational hypertension and pre-eclampsia. Br J Obstet Gynaecol 98: 1239–1244

McLaren M, Greer I A, Walker J J et al 1986 Umbilical artery perfusion: a method to measure prostacyclin production. Prog Lipid Res 25: 311–315

McLaren M, Greer I A, Walker J J et al 1987 Reduced prostacyclin production by umbilical arteries from pregnancy complicated by severe pregnancy induced hypertension. Clin Exp Hypertens B6: 365–374

Marletta M A 1989 Nitric oxide biosynthesis and biological significance. Trends Biochem Sci 14: 488–492

Miller D K, Sandowski S, Soderman D D et al 1985 Endothelial cell prostacyclin production induced by activated neutrophils. J Biol Chem 260: 1006–1014

Moncada S, Palmer R M J, Higgs E A 1991 Nitric oxide: physiology, pathophysiology, and pharmacology. Pharmacol Rev 43: 109–142

Moodley J, Norman R J, Reddi K 1984 Central venous concentrations of immunoreactive prostaglandins E, F and 6-keto-prostaglandin F_1 in eclampsia. Br Med J 288: 1487–1489

Muramatsu M, Iwama Y, Shimizu K et al 1992 Hypoxia-elicited contraction of aorta and coronary artery via removal of endothelium-derived nitric oxide. Am J Physiol 263: H1339–H1347

Myatt L, Brewer A, Brockman D E 1991 The action of nitric oxide in the perfused human fetal–placental circulation. Am J Obstet Gynecol 164: 687–692

Myatt L, Langdon G, Brewer A et al 1992 Characterization of nitric oxide synthase in the human placental villus vascular tree. Society for Gynecologic Investigation 39th annual meeting, San Antonio, Texas, Abstract no. 64

Nova A, Sibai B M, Barton J R et al 1991 Maternal plasma level of endothelin is increased in pre-eclampsia. Am J Obstet Gynecol 165: 724–727

Oian P, Omsjo I, Maltau J M et al 1985 Increased sensitivity to thromboplastin synthesis in blood monocytes from pre-eclamptic patients. Br J Obstet Gynaecol 92: 511–517

Palmer R M J, Ferrige A G, Moncada S 1987 Nitric oxide release accounts for the biological activity of endothelium-derived relaxing factor. Nature 327: 524–526

Phelen J P, Everidge G J, Wilder T L et al 1977 Is the supine pressor test an adequate means of predicting acute hypertension in pregnancy? Am J Obstet Gynecol 128: 173–176

Pijnenborg R, Anthony J, Davey D A, Rees A et al 1991 Placental bed spiral arteries in the hypertensive disorders of pregnancy. Br J Obstet Gynaecol 98: 648–655

Pinto A, Sorrentino R, Sorrentino P et al 1991 Endothelial-derived relaxing factor released by endothelial cells of human umbilical vessels and its impairment in pregnancy-induced hypertension. Am J Obstet Gynecol 164: 507–513

Pologe L G, Cramer E V, Pawlowski N A et al 1984 Stimulation of human endothelial cell prostacyclin synthesis by select leukotrienes. J Exp Med 160: 1043–1053

Rakoczi I, Tallian F, Bagdany S et al 1979 Platelet life-span in normal pregnancy and pre-eclampsia as determined by a non-radioisotope technique. Thromb Results 15: 553–556

Redman C W G, Allington M J, Bolton F G et al 1977a Plasma β-thromboglobulin in pre-eclampsia. Lancet i: 248

Redman C W G, Denson K W E, Beilin L J et al 1977b Factor VIII consumption in pre-eclampsia. Lancet ii: 1249–1252

Redman C W G, Bonnar J, Beilin L J 1978 Early platelet consumption in pre-eclampsia. Br Med J 1: 467–469

Remuzzi G, Misiani R, Muratore D 1979 Prostacyclin and human foetal circulation. Prostaglandins 18: 341–348

Ritter J M, Farquar C, Rodin A et al 1987 Low dose aspirin treatment in late pregnancy differentially inhibits cyclo-oxygenase in maternal platelets. Prostaglandins 34: 717–722

Roberts J M, Taylor R N, Goldfien A 1991 Clinical and biochemical evidence of endothelial cell dysfunction in the pregnancy syndrome preeclampsia. Am J Hypertension 4: 700–708

Rodgers G M, Taylor R N, Roberts J M 1988 Pre-eclampsia is associated with a serum factor cytoxic to human endothelial cells. Am J Obstet Gynecol 159: 908–914

Schiff E, Peleg E, Goldenberg M et al 1989 The use of aspirin to prevent pregnancy-induced hypertension and lower the ratio of thromboxane A_2 to prostaglandin in relatively high risk pregnancies. N Engl J Med 322: 204–205

Schiff E, Barkai G, Ben-Baruch G et al 1990 Low-dose aspirin does not influence the clinical course of women with mild pregnancy-induced hypertension. Obstet Gynecol 76: 742–744

Sibai B M, Mirro R, Chesney C M, Leffler C 1989 Low dose aspirin in pregnancy. Obstet Gynecol 74: 551–557

Sibai B, Caritis C, Phillips E et al 1993 Prevention of preeclampsia: low-dose aspirin in nulliparous women: a double-blind, placebo-controlled trial. Am J Obstet Gynecol 168: 286

Sinzinger H, Virgolini I, Peskar B A 1989 Response of thromboxane B_2 malondialdehyde and platelet sensitivity to 3 weeks low dose aspirin in health volunteers. Thromb Res 53: 261–269

Socol M L, Weiner C P, Louis G et al 1985 Platelet activation in pre-eclampsia. Am J Obstet Gynecol 151: 494–497

Spencer J A D, Smith M J, Cederholm-Williams S A et al 1983 Influence of pre-eclampsia on concentrations of haemostatic factors in mothers and infants. Arch Dis Child 58: 739–741

Stuart M J, Gross S J, Elrad H et al 1982 Effects of acetylsalicylic acid ingestion on maternal and neonatal hemostatis. N Engl J Med 307: 909–912

Suzuki H, Ikenaga H, Hishikawa K et al 1992 Increases in NO_2^-/NO_3^- excretion in the urine as an indicator of the release of endothelium-derived relaxing factor during elevation of blood pressure Clin Sci 82: 631–634

Taylor R N, Casal D C, Jones L A et al 1991 Selective effects of preeclampsia sera on human endothelial cell procoagulant protein expresssion. Am J Obstet Gynecol 165: 1705–1710

Trudinger B J, Stewart G J, Cook C M et al 1988 Monitoring lupus anticoagulant positive pregnancies with umbilical flow velocity waveforms. Obstet Gynecol 72: 215–218

Tulenko T, Schneider J, Floro C et al 1987 The in vitro effect on arterial wall function of serum from patients with pregnancy induced hypertension. Am J Obstet Gynecol 156: 817–823

Tuvemo T 1980 Role of prostaglandins, prostacyclin and thromboxanes in the control of the umbilical–placental circulation. Seminar Perinatol 4: 91–95

Uzan S, Beaufils M, Breart G et al 1991 Prevention of fetal growth retardation with low-dose aspirin: findings of the EPREDA trial. Lancet 337: 1427–1431

Vallance P, Collier J, Moncada S 1989 Effects of endothelium-derived nitric oxide on peripheral arteriolar tone in man. Lancet ii: 997–1000

Wallenburg H C S, Rotmans N 1982 Enhanced reactivity of the platelet thromboxane pathway in normotensive and hypertensive pregnancies with insufficient fetal growth. Am J Obstet Gynecol 144: 523–528

Wallenburg H C S, Rotmans N 1987 Prevention of recurrent idiopathic fetal growth retardation by low-dose aspirin and dipyridamole. Am J Obstet Gynecol 157: 1230–1235

Wallenburg H C S, Dekker G A, Makovitz J W et al 1986 Low dose aspirin prevents pregnancy induced hypertension and pre-eclampsia in angiotensin-sensitive primigravidae. Lancet i: 1–3

Wallenburg H C S, Dekker G A, Makovitz J W et al 1991 Effect of low-dose aspirin on vascular refractoriness in angiotensin-sensitive primigravid women. Am J Obstet Gynecol 164: 1169–1173

Walsh S W 1985 Pre-eclampsia: an imbalance in placental prostacyclin and thromboxane production. Am J Obstet Gynecol 152: 335–340

Warso M A, Lands W E M 1983 Lipid peroxidation in relation to prostacyclin and thromboxane physiology and pathophysiology. Br Med Bull 39: 277–280

2

Recurrent fetal loss and the antiphospholipid syndrome

N. S. Pattison   M. A. Birdsall   L. W. Chamley   W. F. Lubbe

Antiphospholipid antibodies (aPL) comprise a family of autoantibodies which have a well-established association with fetal loss (Harris et al 1988, Branch et al 1985). These antibodies have also been described in association with a variety of medical disorders characterized by thrombocytopenia and/or thrombosis. Recently, successful treatment for women with recurrent fetal loss has been reported (Lubbe et al 1983, Cowchock et al 1992). Despite an exponential increase in the number of publications on aPL, including associations with disease, drugs, diagnostic laboratory tests and characterization of the antibodies, no clear information has emerged on the mechanism of action nor has the optimal therapy for patients with aPL been established.

This chapter will review the prevalence, association, diagnosis and mechanism of action of aPL while focusing on an approach to obstetric management.

ANTIPHOSPHOLIPID SYNDROME

Antiphospholipid antibodies, first detected by Wassermann in 1906, were first described in patients with systemic lupus erythematosus (SLE) by Conley & Hartmann in 1952. Early work suggested an invariable association between the presence of aPL and an underlying connective tissue disorder. As clinical experience has accumulated, it has become clear that most individuals with aPL have no identifiable collagen disorder. The occurrence of a primary antiphospholipid syndrome was proposed by Harris in 1987 consisting of clinical and laboratory features (Table 2.1). Antiphospholipid antibodies are now most commonly described in association with fetal loss, thrombocytopenia or thrombotic events without evidence of autoimmune disease, viz. the antiphospholipid syndrome (APS). The syndrome has become a well-recognized clinical entity.

ANTIPHOSPHOLIPID ANTIBODIES

Antiphospholipid antibodies are a diverse family of autoantibodies which share in common a reactivity with negatively charged phospholipids. There are three clinically significant members.

Table 2.1 Definition of APS
(Must include one clinical and one serological feature)

Clinical features:	Recurrent venous or arterial thrombosis
	Recurrent fetal loss
	Thrombocytopenia
Serological features:	IgG aCL > 20 GPL
	LA
	IgM aCL > 20 MPL plus LA

After Harris (1987).
See text for explanation of abbreviation.

The biological false positive test for syphilis

Serological screening tests for syphilis such as the Venereal Diseases Research Laboratories (VDRL) and rapid plasma reagin (RPR) employ an antigen which is a mixture of phospholipids containing phosphatidyl choline, cholesterol and cardiolipin. The negatively charged cardiolipin (so called because it was originally extracted from bovine heart tissue) reacts with antibodies produced in response to syphilitic infection. These antibodies have been called reagins. Reagins can also be present in the serum of patients who do not have a syphilitic infection and are responsible for the biological false positive test for syphilis (BFP). A BFP can result from:

1. Antibodies produced in response to infection by a number of non-treponemal pathogens (Masala et al 1989). In this situation the BFP is likely to be transient, reflecting recent activity of the pathogen. These antibodies are not associated with thrombosis or fetal loss.
2. Autoantibodies produced by patients with autoimmune diseases, particularly patients with APS and/or SLE. These autoantibodies can persist for many years and are associated with both thrombosis and fetal loss.

Lupus anticoagulant

Lupus anticoagulant (LA) comprises autoantibodies of either IgG or IgM class which prolong phospholipid-dependent coagulation assays by reacting with negatively charged phospholipids (Pengo et al 1987). The name LA is an unfortunate misnomer for two reasons:

1. Although originally found in patients with SLE, LA is more common in patients who do not have this condition.
2. Despite prolonging in vitro coagulation tests, LA have been associated with thrombosis rather than haemorrhage (Shapiro & Thiagarajan 1982).

A number of coagulation assays are currently used to screen for LA. These include the activated partial thromboplastin time (APTT), kaolin clotting time (KCT), dilute Russell viper venom test (dRVVT) and the dilute tissue thromboplastin assay (dTTa) (Triplett & Brandt 1989). There is no agreement in the literature as to which of these tests is most specific or sensitive (Machin et al 1990). It is agreed that no single test can detect all LA.

Anticardiolipin antibodies

The third type of aPL is the anticardiolipin antibody aCL, which is detected by solid-phase immunoassay (enzyme-linked immunosorbent assay (ELISA) or radioimmunoassay (RIA)) (Harris et al 1983, Pattison et al 1987). Historically, the aCL assay may be considered to be a development from the RPR and VDRL for syphilis which utilize a cardiolipin antigen. It was noted that patients with LA often had a BFP test for syphilis. It was reasoned that the same antibody was causing both the BFP and LA reactions but that the BFP lacked the sensitivity to detect all LA. The aCL assay has proved to be 200–400 times more sensitive than the VDRL test and detected 91% of the LA in the original population studied (Harris et al 1983).

Antibodies to other phospholipids

Phospholipid antigens other than cardiolipin have been used in solid-phase assays for aPL because cardiolipin is unlikely to be the physiological antigen for aCL as it is found almost exclusively in the mitochondria and is not exposed to circulating aPL (Hecht 1965).

Phosphatidyl serine (PS) has been used as an alternative antigen as most aCL will bind to PS which, unlike cardiolipin, is located in membranes of endothelial cells and platelets. However, PS is found in the interior leaflet of non-activated cell membranes and is only exposed to circulating antibodies after cell activation causes its transfer to the exterior leaflet. Thus there is some question as to whether PS can be the physiological antigen for aPL. Other laboratories test for antibodies to phosphatidyl ethanolamine, which is present in both the interior and exterior leaflets of cell membranes and thus is exposed to circulating aPL.

The anticardiolipin antibody cofactor, β_2-glycoprotein 1

The requirement of a cofactor to facilitate the binding of aCL to phospholipids has been described recently (Galli et al 1990a, McNeil et al 1990, Matsuura et al 1990, Chamley et al 1991a). The cofactor, which is present in normal serum, has been identified as β_2-glycoprotein 1 (β_2-GP1; also called apolipoprotein H) (McNeil et al 1990). The in vivo role β_2-GP1 is unknown but this role may reflect the in vitro properties of β_2-GP1 which are:

1. An inhibitor of the intrinsic phase of coagulation
2. An inhibitor of platelet activation

3. A phospholipid binding protein (Wurm 1984, Schousboe 1985, Nimpf et al 1987).

Possibly the formation of a trimolecular complex involving β_2-GP1, aCL and phospholipid prevents the normal function of β_2-GP1. In light of this suggestion it is interesting to note that Matsuura et al (1990) have demonstrated that, unlike aCL of autoimmune origin, aCL resulting from syphilitic or other infections bind to phospholipid in the absence of β_2-GP1. This difference in the cofactor requirements of aCL from various origins may explain why only aCL of autoimmune origin are associated with thrombosis and recurrent fetal loss.

Interrelationship of antiphospholipid antibody subtypes

The three aPL(BFP, LA and aCL) were originally thought to be different manifestations of the same antibody. However, recent reports of the chromatographic separation of these antibodies from each other (Exner et al 1988, McNeil et al 1988, Chamley et al 1991b) plus the incomplete concordance of these antibodies in studies with unselected populations suggest that in the majority of cases these are different antibodies (Branch et al 1987, Hazeline et al 1988). However, it is possible that some antibodies could express all three aPL activities (Fig. 2.1).

All three aPL (LA, aCL and BPS) are independently associated with fetal loss. Yet many women with these antibodies do not suffer fetal loss. The question remains: is there an antibody yet to be discovered for which the current group of aPL (LA, aCL and BPS) are markers?

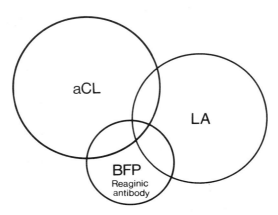

Fig. 2.1   Venn diagram demonstrating a possible interrelationship of antiphospholipid antibody subtypes.

DIAGNOSTIC TESTS FOR ANTIPHOSPHOLIPID ANTIBODIES

Biological false positive test for syphilis

The BFP reaction requires:

1. That a phospholipid-based screening assay such as the VDRL is persistently positive (for 6 months)
2. That the absence of treponemal infection is confirmed by a non-phospholipid-based assay such as the TPHA (Schulman 1987).

Lupus anticoagulant

The minimal criteria for the detection of LA proposed by Triplett & Brandt (1989) are:

1. A prolongation of a phospholipid-dependent screening test such as the APTT
2. Demonstration that the abnormality is due to an inhibitor (rather than a factor deficiency)
3. Proof that the inhibitor is directed against phospholipids (Triplett & Brandt 1989).

Screening tests

The most common of the screening tests for LA is the APTT. In this assay an activator and a phospholipid mixture (partial thromboplastin) trigger the contact phase of coagulation in the plasma sample. LA will bind to the phospholipid and prolong the assay. A variety of APTT reagents are available, each of which differs in phospholipid content and sensitivity to LA. Thus APTT results may vary greatly from one laboratory to another.

The KCT, devised by Exner et al (1978), is used to screen for LA by many laboratories in Australasia and Europe. In this system the contact phase of coagulation is activated by the addition of kaolin. No exogenous phospholipid is added, making this test very sensitive to LA (Lesperance et al 1988). However, any phospholipid contamination will adversely affect this assay. A second major disadvantage of the KCT is that it is laborious and cannot be automated.

The dRVVT is also widely used as a screening assay for LA and has a similar sensitivity to the KCT (Creagh & Greaves 1991). This assay utilizes a snake venom with a mixture of phospholipid to activate factor X. Thus it is less prone to detect factor deficiencies than other assays. Like the APTT the dRVVT suffers from variability due to different reagents (Brandt & Triplett 1989).

Demonstration of an inhibitor

In order to confirm the presence of an inhibitor the screening test is repeated using a mixture (usually 1 : 1) of the patient's plasma with a normal plasma. If the abnormality is due to an inhibitor the test will remain prolonged. If the abnormality is due to a factor deficiency the normal plasma will act as a source of the factor and the test result will correct to normal.

Proof that the inhibitor is directed against phospholipid

A platelet neutralization procedure (PNP) is used to confirm the antiphospholipid nature of an inhibitor. Lysed platelets are added to the abnormal plasma, and the screening test (APTT or dRVVT) is repeated. An abnormality caused by LA will correct in a PNP whilst an abnormality due to a factor inhibitor will not.

Pre-analytical variables

Sample preparation is critical for accurate measurement of LA. This is because any cellular debris (phospholipid) will bind to mask the presence of LA, thus:

1. Any degree of haemolysis is unacceptable
2. It is desirable to remove the plasma from the whole blood as soon after collection as possible to avoid cell lysis
3. Samples must be double centrifuged or filtered to ensure platelet removal.

Anticardiolipin antibodies

Anticardiolipin antibodies are most frequently detected by ELISA. In this system purified cardiolipin is coated onto the wells of a plastic ELISA plate. Patients' serum is then diluted and added to the wells. If the serum contains aCL these will bind to the cardiolipin and the unbound serum is then washed off. A second antibody which recognizes human IgG or IgM is then added. This second antibody will bind to any aCL which is present. The second antibody carries an enzyme label which will produce a colour change when added to its substrate. Thus the amount of aCL in a sample is determined by the amount of colour change in the ELISA. Unlike the LA assays the aCL ELISA employs serum which requires no special treatment. Up to 50 samples can be assayed on each ELISA plate. Anticardiolipin antibody ELISAs are subject to excessive inter-laboratory variability (Peaceman et al 1992). Although many factors may contribute to this variability, it has long been known that the sample diluent used in the assay is critical (Harris et al 1987). Only assays utilizing bovine serum as the diluent are reliable. This is due to the requirement of the aCL cofactor which is present in bovine serum but absent from other routinely used diluents (Chamley et al 1991a). A second hurdle to the usefulness of the aCL assay is the continued failure of the international community to agree on a standard unit for reporting test results. This is despite the availability of standards from an international standardization workshop [Kingston Anti-Phospholipid Antibody Study (KAPS)] which utilize the units GPL and MPL. One MPL or GPL unit is equivalent to $1\mu g$ of affinity-purified aCL, IgM or IgG (Harris 1990).

PREVALENCE OF ANTIPHOSPHOLIPID ANTIBODIES

The prevalence of aPL in the general population is unclear. A small study has indicated that the prevalence of LA is 3.6% and of aCL 4–6% (Shi et al 1990).

Prevalence in the obstetric population

The prevalence of aPL, both LA and aCL, in the general obstetric population is approximately 2% (Table 2.2). This range of reported prevalences of aPL reflects disagreement in cut-off levels for test positivity, population selection, variation in assay methods and accuracy. If a low cut-off level is chosen the prevalence is high but association with fetal loss less strong. Indeed one of the four large population studies did not find an association with fetal deaths (Harris & Spinnato 1992). It also remains unclear in what percentage of women aCL and/or LA tests are positive during pregnancy yet negative between pregnancies.

A population study in 1987 of 1000 consecutively booked antenatal patients at the National Women's Hospital, Auckland, revealed the overall prevalence of aPL to be 1.9%, with aCL found in 1% (9 women) and LA in 1.2% (11 women) of the population (2 women had both antibodies) (Pattison et al 1993). In this study 2 of the women with LA had fetal losses, and a further 4 had adverse pregnancy outcomes. Five had normal pregnancies. Five of the 9 women with aCL had complicated pregnancies; 3 miscarried and 2 had pre-eclampsia. Four women had a normal outcome. The presence of aPL correlated with adverse pregnancy outcome.

Lockwood et al (1989) studied 737 consecutively enrolled obstetric women and found a prevalence of 2% for aPL. The prevalence of LA was 2.7/1000 and for aCL 22/1000. In their study population 100% of women with LA experienced mid-trimester fetal loss and 75% of women with aCL experi-

Table 2.2 Prevalence data from normal obstetric populations

No. of subjects	Prevalence (%) aCL	LA	Percentage with fetal loss	Authors
737	2.2	0.2	75%	Lockwood et al (1989)
1200	1.25[a]	—	NIL	Perez et al (1991)
1200	0.5[b]		50%	Perez et al (1991)
1449	6.2	—	No adverse outcomes	Harris & Spinnato (1992)
1000	1.0	1.2	17%	Pattison et al (1992)

[a]Low titre.
[b]High titre.

enced an adverse pregnancy outcome (perinatal loss, preterm delivery or IUGR); thus the presence of aCL or LA was strongly correlated with an adverse obstetric outcome.

Perez and his colleagues (1991) confirmed these findings in an obstetric population of 1200 women. Low levels of IgG were present in 1.25% of women but these were not associated with an adverse outcome. Of the 0.5% of women who had a moderate or high level of IgG, 50% experienced a fetal loss.

In a study of 1447 pregnant women at term the overall prevalence of aPL was 6% (Harris & Spinnato 1992). The majority of these (78 of 89) were low positive results, detected by the newer and more sensitive assays. Only 3 women had medium levels (>20 GPL units); 1.79% of the population was positive for IgG, and 4.3% were positive for IgM. Anticardiolipin positivity did not correlate with pregnancy complications or outcome in this population, possibly reflecting the low titre taken as a cut-off for positivity and/or the IgM fraction. These low levels are thought to be of less clinical significance. However, by studying a population at term, early fetal loss, a major complication of aPL, was automatically excluded.

Prevalence of aPL in patients with SLE

A meta-analysis of 29 reported series which comprises over 1000 patients with SLE revealed the prevalence of LA to be 34% and 44% for aCL (Love & Santoro 1989). A definite correlation between the presence of aCL and LA was found; among patients with SLE and LA, 59% will have aCL, and 45% of patients with SLE and aCL will have LA.

Prevalence in selected populations of pregnant women

The conclusion from these population studies is that the prevalence of aPL in a normal obstetric population is low — approximately 2%. The prevalence in selected populations with fetal loss is significantly higher. There does appear to be an association between antibody presence and adverse pregnancy outcome. However, not all women with aPL will have complicated pregnancies. The correlation with adverse pregnancy outcome is best with higher levels of LA or aCL; however, a better predictor of adverse outcome is a previous fetal loss. In the above studies 50% of women with aPL had a normal outcome and therapy does not seem to be indicated for this group.

There have been a number of retrospective studies confirming an association between antibody presence and fetal loss. Three selected groups of pregnant women have been studied, as discussed below.

Women with recurrent miscarriage

Recurrent first trimester miscarriage is the commonest clinical scenario in women with aPL. Various authors have found the incidence of aPL in women with three or more first trimester miscarriages to vary between 14% (Barbui et al 1988) and 42% (Unander et al 1987).

Many groups have studied patients attending hospital and recurrent miscarriage clinics and found an increased incidence of aPL when compared with the normal obstetric population. Creagh et al (1991) investigated 66 women; 31 had experienced one or two pregnancy losses and 35 had had three or more pregnancy losses. In the first group 10% had aPL; one woman was positive for LA, none were positive for aCL IgG and two were positive for aCL IgM. In the second group with three or more recurrent miscarriages, 31% had aPL; 7 were positive for LA, 1 for aCL IgG and 3 for aCL IgM. These authors concluded that LA and aCL IgG are independent risk factors for fetal loss. Parke et al (1991) compared three groups of women: women with recurrent miscarriage, women who had undergone normal pregnancy and women who had never been pregnant. They found a positive frequency of aPL in 16%, 7% and 3%, respectively. In a study of women in this institution with recurrent miscarriage 41% (33/81) had aPL, usually at low level (Birdsall et al 1992).

Women with later fetal death

Late fetal losses are also associated with aPL. Toyoshima and colleagues (1991) in their group of 104 patients with recurrent fetal loss found that 42.8% of patients with late fetal losses were positive for aCL. Twenty-nine per cent (18/60) of normally formed stillbirths delivering in this institution from 1989 to 1991 were associated with aPL (Birdsall et al 1992).

Case–control studies

There have been two case-control studies drawing opposing conclusions. Parazzini et al (1991) examined the association between aPL and pregnancy outcome in 220 women with a history of recurrent miscarriage and compared them with 193 controls. They found that 7% of the women with a history of recurrent miscarriage were positive for LA; no patient in the control group had LA. Nineteen per cent of women with recurrent miscarriage were positive for aCL versus 3% of controls ($p < 0.001$). In contrast, Infante-Rivard (1991) and colleagues conducted a case–control study of 331 women with a single spontaneous miscarriage or fetal death and 993 controls without previous spontaneous fetal loss. These authors found LA in 5.1% of cases and 3.8% of controls — a non-significant difference. Anticardiolipin was present in 1.2% of cases and 1.5% of controls. These authors concluded that there is no apparent justification for considering aPL to be a risk factor for fetal loss among women who present with spontaneous miscarriage or fetal death and have no previous spontaneous fetal loss. This study contrasts strikingly with other reports, and suffers from the disadvantage that all the cases had only had one miscarriage, where the incidence of antibody positivity would be expected to be low. Any positive results would be vastly diluted by the number of non-recurrent miscarriages.

Two authors have addressed the question of whether LA or aCL correlates better with adverse outcome. Lockshin (1990) noted that fetal death occurred in 77% (10 of 13) women with SLE with aCL alone versus 50% (6 of 12) patients with LA alone. He concluded that aCL was more sensitive and specific for predicting fetal death than LA. However, a prospective study by Pattison et al (1992) suggested that elevated levels of aCL and the presence of LA have equal predictive values for a poor obstetric outcome.

PATHOGENESIS

The prime area of focus in pregnancies complicated by aPL has been the placenta and the underlying decidual vessels. A wide range of placental appearances have been reported, from the normal, to the small infarcted placenta, to those with extensive atherosis (Hanley et al 1988).

A number of workers have demonstrated the failure of the normal physiological adaptation to pregnancy. In the non-pregnant uterus the spiral arteries supplying the endometrium are narrow, muscular-walled vessels. Upon implantation the endometrium is converted to decidua. Placental cytotrophoblast invades the spiral arteries, replacing the endothelial cell lining and destroying the muscular and elastic tissue of the vessel walls. This allows these vessels to accommodate the increased blood flow required during pregnancy. This metamorphosis is called the 'physiological changes of pregnancy' (Brossens et al 1967). Antiphospholipid antibodies may prevent these physiological changes of pregnancy (Fig. 2.2).

Histological examination shows abnormalities in the decidual vessels. These vessels commonly show a vasculopathy where there is fibrinoid necrosis and an inflammatory cell infiltrate with decidual necrosis (De Wolf et al 1982) (Fig. 2.3). Immunofluorescence studies demonstrate a large deposition of immunoglobulin in the walls of the decidual vessels. These appearances have recently been elegantly replicated in an animal model by Branch et al (1990). Mice were injected with the IgG fraction of serum containing aPL, resulting in a fetal loss. Histological examination of the uteroplacental interface showed decidual necrosis, and immunofluorescent studies demonstrated prominent intravascular IgG and fibrin deposition. These pathological appearances could well account for the spectrum of clinical disease seen in the obstetric patient with aPL. The early fetal losses may be secondary to inadequate maternal blood supply through the diseased decidual vessels, culminating in fetal hypoxia with subsequent loss. Later losses or growth retardation may be a less severe manifestation of this process.

It is unknown whether a decidual vasculopathy is the primary event or whether thrombosis occurring in either the decidual vessels or intervillous spaces causes subsequent changes in the vessel walls. More work is needed to

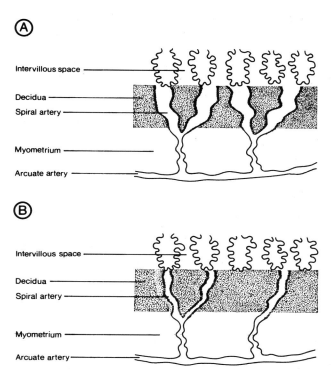

Fig. 2.2 Diagrammatic representation of possible explanation for vasculopathy associated with antiphospholipid antibodies. **A** Normal physiological adaptation to pregnancy. **B** Maladaptation with lack of vasodilatation and reduced vessel number.

elucidate the exact nature and chronology of events in pregnancies complicated by aPL.

MECHANISM OF ACTION OF ANTIPHOSPHOLIPID ANTIBODIES

At present the mechanism of action of aPL in the clinical situation is unknown. Investigations are continuing on several putative mechanisms. The work on these mechanisms of action of aPL is summarized below.

Effect on platelets

Early workers described thrombocytopenia as a frequent finding in patients with aPL (Harris et al 1985). This finding coupled to the thrombotic nature of APS prompted the suggestion that aPL may bind to and disrupt the function of platelet membrane phospholipids. However, phospholipids are distributed asymmetrically in the non-activated platelet membrane. The negatively charged phospholipids, with which aPL react, are present only in

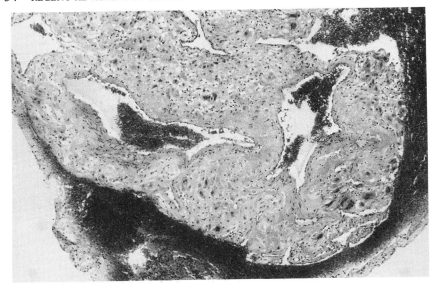

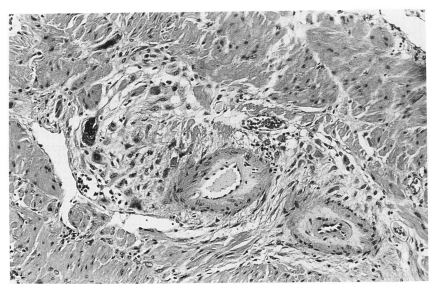

Fig. 2.3 Histological section of placenta. **A** Normal physiological change to a decidual vessel. **B** Failed response in the presence of antiphospholipid antibodies.

the inner leaflet (Gerrard & Friesen 1985). Therefore, non-activated platelets should not be antigenic for aPL. Upon activation the distribution of phospholipids in the platelet membrane is altered with the transfer of the negatively charged PS to the exterior leaflet of the membrane. This permits the platelet to participate in the processes of coagulation and may make them antigenic for aPL. Khamashta et al (1988) confirmed the inability of aPL to react with non-activated platelets but demonstrated the binding of these antibodies to disrupted platelets where the inner leaflet had been exposed. Thus platelets must be activated to facilitate aPL binding and it is unlikely that aPL cause thrombosis by inducing platelet activation.

Effect on the vascular endothelium

The vascular endothelium plays a pivotal role in the maintenance of normal haemostasis. Several groups have demonstrated the coexistence of aPL and anti-endothelial cell antibodies in the serum of patients with SLE or APS (Cines et al 1984, Carvera et al 1991). Of the haemostatic functions of the endothelial cell, three may be disrupted by aPL.

Inhibition of prostacyclin production

Prostacyclin, a potent vasodilator, is produced in endothelial cells by a pathway which requires the release of arachidonic acid from the phospholipids of the cell membrane by phospholipase A_2 (Fig. 2.4). It has been proposed that aPL which react with membrane phospholipid would inhibit the production of prostacyclin by the vascular endothelium and promote thrombosis (Carreras et al 1981b). In support of this hypothesis Carreras et al (1981) demonstrated that the IgG fraction from the serum of a patient with LA could inhibit the production of prostacyclin by rat aortic rings and human myometrium (Carreras et al 1981a). This decrease in prostacyclin formation was reversed by the addition of free arachidonic acid, suggesting that the LA was inhibiting the release of arachidonic acid from membrane phospholipid (Fig. 2.4) (Carreras et al 1981a). Despite early enthusiasm for

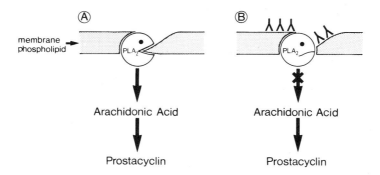

Fig. 2.4   A model for the inhibition of phospholipase A_2 (PLA$_2$) by aPL. **A** Normal release of arachidonic acid by PLA$_2$. **B** The binding of aPL (λ) to cell membrane could disrupt arachidonic acid release inhibiting prostaglandin synthesis.

this mechanism of action and some confirmatory studies (Schorer et al 1989), numerous workers have been unable to duplicate these results (Hasselaar et al 1988, Rustin et al 1988). Whilst it now seems unlikely that reduction in the production of prostacyclin by endothelial cells is the sole cause of aPL-mediated thrombosis this mechanism may contribute to thrombosis in some individuals.

Inactivation of the protein C/protein S/thrombomodulin pathway

Protein C acts as an anticoagulant by inhibiting the activated coagulation factors Va, VIIIa and the platelet bound Va–Xa complex (Kwaan 1989). Two steps in this pathway are phospholipid dependent and may be inhibited by aPL:

1. Protein C is activated by thrombomodulin—a protein present on the surface of vascular endothelial cells. Thrombomodulin must be bound to phospholipid to yield optimum protein C activation (Freyssinet et al 1986). Several authors have demonstrated that aPL can inhibit the in vitro activation of protein C by thrombomodulin (Freyssinet et al 1986, Tsakiris et al 1990).

2. Once activated, protein C requires a cofactor, designated protein S, which facilitates the binding of activated protein C to the platelet membrane (Comp 1990). Once bound to the platelet membrane, the protein C/protein S complex then inhibits coagulation factors Va and Xa. Several groups have demonstrated that aPL can interact with phospholipids and inhibit the protein S-dependent anticoagulant activity of activated protein C (Marcinak et al 1989).

Other studies have failed to detect an inhibitory effect of aPL on the protein C pathway, and it is suggested that inhibition of this pathway could be a mechanism by which aPL cause thrombosis in a limited group of patients (Oosting et al 1992).

Inhibition of the antithrombin III anticoagulant pathway

Endothelial cells express upon their surface heparin-like molecules — glycosaminoglycans (GAGs) — which activate antithrombin III (ATIII) (Andersson 1979). The GAG heparan sulphate is believed to be the physiological activator of ATIII and is particularly important as an anticoagulant in the microcirculation (Marcum et al 1986). Galli et al (1990b) examined the proposition that aPL could cross-react with GAGs and inhibit the activation of ATIII. These workers investigated aPL affinity purified from the serum of four patients and were unable to find any such cross-reactive antibodies. However, a larger study performed in this laboratory demonstrated that 11% of patients with aPL have antibodies which cross-react with heparin and can inhibit the activation of ATIII (Chamley et al 1993). Thus inhibition of GAG-dependent ATIII activity may also be a mechanism of action for

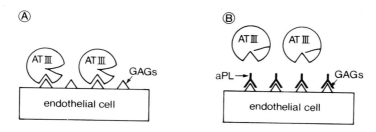

Fig. 2.5 A model for the inhibition of ATIII by aPL. The binding of cross-reactive aPL to endothelial cell GAGs could prevent the potentiation of ATIII by these molecules. **A** Binding of ATIII to endothelial GAGs potentiates this anticoagulant. **B** Binding of cross-reactive aPL to the endothelial GAGs may prevent the binding of ATIII.

some aPL (Fig. 2.5).

No one single pathogenetic mechanism of action for aPL has been identified, but a number of different mechanisms may operate, each of which can explain the activity of some aPL. This is not surprising when it is considered that aPL are an extremely diverse family of antibodies.

CLINICAL ASSOCIATIONS

The hallmark of the presence of aPL is the triad of arterial and venous thrombosis, thrombocytopenia and fetal loss. It remains unclear whether these disease entities are associations or direct pathological consequences of the presence of aPL. Even though it has become increasingly common to measure these antibodies in the evaluation of patients with a history of unexplained reproductive failure, the significance of knowing a patient's antibody status independent of her clinical history remains unknown.

Medical disorders

The medical manifestations, first recognized in patients with aPL, were related to arterial or venous thrombosis involving virtually any vascular bed, e.g. deep venous thrombosis with pulmonary embolism, retinal arterial or venous thrombosis, renal, mesenteric or coeliac vascular occlusion, thrombotic stroke and upper limb vascular occlusion. It is now recognized that the spectrum of aPL-related disorders stretches far wider and includes other thrombotic disorders. Neurological disorders such as transient ischaemic attacks, amaurosis fugax, migraine-like headaches, acute ischaemic encephalopathy, multi-infarct dementia and degenerative myelopathy are now recognized as representing aPL-related phenomena. Cardiac disorders associated with the aPL syndrome include valvular lesions, valvular or chamber thrombosis and coronary artery occlusion. Adrenal gland involvement by vascular occlusion may manifest as Addison's disease. A thrombotic vasculopathy may involve the vessels of skin (livedo reticularis) or lungs. Lung disease may result in the development of pulmonary hypertension with histological features resembling primary pulmonary hypertension. Snedden's syndrome comprises the clinical triad of livedo reticularis, cerebrovascular occlusion and labile hypertension in the presence of aPL (Schulze-Lohoft et al 1989).

Neither the type (IgG or IgM) nor the level of aPL can be used to identify individuals prone to future thrombotic episodes. Prolonged periods of follow-up have indicated infrequent change in the level or type of antibody in the majority of individuals (Asherson et al 1991).

Anticardiolipin antibodies of the IgM isotype are frequently found following acute infections such as mycoplasma, adenovirus, rubella, chickenpox, mumps, Epstein–Barr virus, parvovirus, Gram-negative infections and latterly human immunodeficiency virus. Drugs such as procainamide, quinidine, phenytoin, chlorpromazine, valproic acid, amoxycillin, hydrallazine and propranolol have also been reported to induce aPL. These drug-induced aPL are generally not associated with thrombotic complications or fetal loss.

From various surveys it appears that 30–50% of individuals with SLE also have aPL. Evidence for an underlying collagen disorder can be found in 30–40% of individuals with aPL.

Obstetric disorders

In 1975 Nilsson and co-workers first made the observation that aPL may be associated with recurrent fetal loss. They described an apparently healthy young woman who suffered three unexpected late fetal deaths. All were associated with placental infarction and abruption. She later went on to suffer deep venous thrombosis and pulmonary emboli. An inhibitor of thromboplastin generation was identified in her plasma.

Antiphospholipid antibodies are associated with fetal loss and pregnancy complications.

Fetal loss

There are three patterns of fetal loss observed in women with aPL:

1. First trimester miscarriage
2. Later fetal loss with evidence of growth retardation
3. Later fetal loss without evidence of growth retardation.

First trimester miscarriage can be both very early (prior to detection of fetal heart activity on ultrasound) or following confirmation of fetal presence. They are not clinically different from spontaneous miscarriages.

In women with later fetal losses complicated by growth retardation the placenta is generally small, with multiple infarcts and calcification. These pregnancies have often been associated with early-onset gestational proteinuric hypertension. Frequently a patient with a history of recurrent first trimester miscarriage will develop these complications in the mid or early third trimester in a subsequent pregnancy.

When later losses are observed in the absence of growth retardation, the placenta may be of normal size and may or may not show evidence of infarcts. Investigation of so-called unexplained fetal death will frequently detect aPL.

Other obstetric complications

Those pregnancies in women with aPL which do not end in fetal loss, have a high incidence of other obstetric complications which may reflect the spectrum of pathogenicity seen with these antibodies (Table 2.3). Severe second trimester gestational proteinuric hypertension (GPH) associated with growth retardation is a common event in women with aPL. Branch et al (1989) reported on 43 women with GPH and found that 16% (7 of 43) had significant levels of aPL. Of those 7, significant maternal morbidity occurred in the peripartum period, with cerebral infarction, pulmonary embolism and transient monocular blindness and amnesia being reported. The more usual late-onset GPH in the 'well' primigravid is generally not associated with aPL.

Table 2.3   Obstetric complications observed in women with antiphospholipid antibodies

Recurrent first trimester miscarriage
Fetal death
Intrauterine growth retardation
Placental abruption
Pre-eclampsia — often severe and early onset
Chorea gravidarum

Placental abruption continues to be a significant cause of obstetric mortality and morbidity. Birdsall et al (1992) found that 33% (7/21) women who had a stillbirth due to placental abruption had aPL.

SCREENING

Recognition of the associations between pregnancy complications and aPL has led to investigation of women with recurrent fetal loss and/or adverse pregnancy outcome for the presence of aPL. It is our recommendation that high-risk groups are screened to identify aetiology and to increase treatment options (Table 2.4). The separate identity of LA and aCL means both LA and aCL tests must be negative before aPL can be excluded as a cause for clinical symptoms.

Table 2.4   Indications for investigation of the presence of antiphospholipid antibodies in an obstetric population

---

All autoimmune diseases
Thrombocytopenia
Previous arterial or venous thrombotic event
BFP VDRL
Recurrent (⩾ 3) first trimester miscarriages
All fetal losses after 20 weeks of pregnancy
Placental abruption (previous or current pregnancy)
Fetal growth retardation (previous or current pregnancy)
Severe early-onset pre-eclampsia (previous or current pregnancy)
Chorea gravidarum

MANAGEMENT

General

The presence of aPL confers a high degree of risk to both the woman and her fetus. Referral to a tertiary care centre where expertise in perinatology, haematology and immunological medicine is available is essential. Active involvement by a physician with an interest in obstetrics is highly desirable.

Care of the mother

Not only is the woman with APS at significant risk of hypertension, venous thrombosis, pulmonary embolism or thrombocytopenia, but she may also develop activation of her autoimmune disease. These patients require careful and frequent assessment.

At booking patients with APS and medical sequelae should have a formal assessment by a physician. Particular care must be taken to assess the severity of her disease — measuring the level of target organ damage related to hypertension, renal involvement, thrombocytopenia and activity of her autoimmune disease. Biochemical indices of renal function and serum complement levels should be obtained as baseline observations.

Women with moderate or high-level aCL or LA and without systemic disease should be reviewed each trimester by an obstetric physician. The level of LA or aCL should be checked monthly, and if the KCT is prolonged reconsideration should be given to pharmacological treatment.

Woman with low-level LA or aCL without evidence of autoimmune disease, hypertension or renal disease can be managed by an obstetrician alone. As well as usual antenatal care these patients require regular assessment to detect any medical sequelae, including questioning into joint or systemic symptoms. Platelet count, LA and aCL should be measured on a bimonthly basis.

Care of the fetus

Surveillance offered depends on the past obstetric history. A first trimester ultrasound scan before treatment is commenced is essential to ensure viability and for accurate dating. For those with recurrent first trimester miscarriage, once fetal viability has been confirmed and therapy initiated, there is value in the reassurance and support of a recurrent miscarriage clinic. Frequently these patients will have complications later in pregnancy and require management as below.

Later management for the above patients and those with mid- and third trimester complications in previous pregnancies is aimed at the early detection of the complications associated with aPL — fetal growth retardation, gestational proteinuric hypertension and placental abruption. The patient should be counselled about the importance of not smoking and of regular clinic attendance. Education about the symptoms of preterm labour, placental abruption and fetal movements should be given. In our institution a fetal movement chart is provided from 24 weeks gestation and monthly ultrasound scans obtained from 20 weeks for the early detection of growth retardation. Once growth retardation is detected, usual obstetric management for the unit should be initiated. It is the practice in our institution to monitor fetal growth fortnightly with ultrasound once growth retardation is detected and for women with abnormal Doppler flow studies twice-weekly clinic visits including cardiotocograph (CTG) and/or biophysical profiles. Women with normal Doppler studies are assessed weekly as above. If the pregnancy is progressing normally we would await the onset of spontaneous labour.

Specific therapy

The optimum therapy for women with APS remains uncertain and, indeed, whether any specific therapy is necessary is unclear. While the presence of aPL does confer a risk for pregnancy there have been many reports of successful outcome without treatment (Lockshin et al 1989). The particularly heterogeneous nature of these antibodies, combined with the lack of controlled therapeutic trials to date, makes treatment decisions difficult and this is compounded by the need for caution when treating any pregnant women with medication. It is the practice in our institution to base treatment on past obstetric history. For patients with a past history of fetal loss or pregnancy complications and aPL, specific therapy is recommended. For primigravid women with aPL, after full discussion we recommend close observation without specific therapy.

Successful pregnancy outcomes have been reported using corticosteroids, aspirin, heparin, warfarin, azathiaprine, plasmapheresis, immunoglobulin or combinations of the above. None will guarantee a livebirth. Only one randomized controlled trial is reported in the literature to date — that of Cowchock et al (1992), who compared heparin and aspirin with corticosteroids and aspirin; a placebo group was not included. Table 2.5 gives further details.

Table 2.5 Pregnancy outcome using various therapies

A Single-agent therapy

1. Corticosteroids

Mechanism of action: immune suppression by inhibiting the production of interleukin 2 by T4 cells

Dosage: 40–60 mg per day—reduced when KCT value decreases

Side-effects: Cushingoid features, acne, adrenal insufficiency, diabetes mellitus, oral candida, hypertension, osteoporosis

Reported literature	No. of Pregnancies	Outcome
Carreras et al (1972)	1	1 stillbirth
Hartikalnen-Sorri et al (1980)	1	1 livebirth
Ros et al (1983)	3	3 livebirths
Claurel et al (1986)	3	3 miscarriages
Hedfors et al (1987)	1	1 miscarriage
Overall livebirth rate: 44% (4/9)		

2. Heparin

Mechanism of action: facilitates the action of ATIII

Dosage: subcutaneous heparin sufficient to increase APTT to 1.5–2.0 times normal in those with normal APTT, or if APTT prolonged already heparin dose sufficient to achieve thrombin time of >100 s

Side-effects: bruising, thrombocytopenia, osteoporosis, bleeding

Reported literature	No. of Pregnancies	Outcome
Rosove et al (1990)	15	14 livebirths
Lubbe & Pattison (1991)	1	1 livebirth
Helgren, et al (1982)	9	5 miscarriages, 4 livebirths
Gardlund (1984)	1	1 livebirth
Overall livebirth rate: 77% (20/26)		

3. Aspirin

Mechanism of action: inhibits cyclooxygenase in the platelet which preferentially lowers platelet thromboxane, leaving endothelial prostacyclin synthesis relatively intact

Dosage: 75–80 mg per day

Side-effects: Nil significant reported

Reported literature	No. of Pregnancies	Outcome
Lubbe & Pattison (1991)	12	10 livebirths
Overall livebirth rate: 83% (10/12)		

Table 2.5 Pregnancy outcome using various therapies (*contd*)

B Combination therapy
1. Corticosteroids plus low-dose aspirin
Most commonly reported combination
Usual dosages used as outlined in aspirin and steroid sections

Reported literature	No. of Pregnancies	Outcome
Ordi et al (1989)	9	7 livebirths
Lubbe and Pattison (1991)	31	25 livebirths, 4 miscarriages
Branch et al (1991)	38	25 livebirths
Norberg et al (1987)	5	5 livebirths
Reece et al (1989)	18	14 livebirths, 3 miscarriages, 1 late miscarriage
Blumenfeld et al (1991)	17	15 livebirths, 1 neonatal death
Farquharson et al (1984)	2	2 livebirths, 2 miscarriages
Lockshin et al (1989)[a]	2	14 livebirths
Gatenby (1989)	27	17 livebirths

Overall livebirth rate: 68% (114/168)

[a]Dose of steroids was lower than in other studies — usually <30 mg per day — and duration of treatment was shorter.
[b]If Lockshin's study is removed: 75% (110/147).

2. Heparin plus low-dose aspirin

Reported literature	No. of Pregnancies	Outcome
Branch et al (1990)	8	8 livebirths
Cowchock (1990)	8	6 livebirths

Overall livebirth rate: 88% (14/16)

3. Azathioprine plus corticosteroid
Mechanism of action: acts as an immune suppressant by purine antimetabolism
Dosage of azathioprine used: 75–100 mg
Side-effects: bone marrow depression

Reported literature	No. of Pregnancies	Outcome
Ros et al (1983)	2	1 livebirth
Lockshin (1985)	25	17 livebirths
Gregonni (1986)	1	1 livebirth

Overall livebirth rate: 68% (19/28)

4. Immunoglobulin prednisone plus low-dose aspirin

Reported literature	No. of Pregnancies	Outcome
Scott et al (1988)	1	1 livebirth
Lubbe & Pattison (1991)	3	3 livebirths
Branch et al (1991)	3	1 livebirth

Overall livebirth rate: 71% (5/7)

Contd on p. 44

Table 2.5 Pregnancy outcome using various therapies (*contd*)

C. Controlled trial
1. Heparin plus low-dose aspirin versus corticosteroid plus low-dose aspirin (Cowchock et al (1992)

	Heparin	Corticosteroid
Number	9	6
Livebirth	75%	75%
Preterm delivery*	2	6
Preterm rupture of membranes*	0	3
Mean gestation (weeks)*	37	32
GPH*	0	3

*$P < 0.05$.

CURRENT PRACTICE

The current approach to patients with APS in our institution is to base therapy on past obstetric history and to minimize pharmacological therapy (Fig. 2.6).

Women with antiphospholipid antibodies without previous loss or significant medical disease

There is no evidence that these patients require therapy. Population studies show that most women with low positive aCL or LA have a normal outcome. The question for the primigravid woman is, of course, unknown. Our current practice is to provide these patients with careful monitoring alone.

Antiphospholipid syndrome with fetal loss

Low-level antibodies (aCL < 60 GPL; KCT < 250 s). For these women clinical practice is based on their past obstetric history. All patients in this group require close supervision for both mother and fetus as described above. However, many patients with low-level antibodies will deliver a normally grown infant at term without intervention. Therefore, pharmacological intervention with drugs with significant side-effects is not warranted. There are no placebo-controlled trials to help us with this decision and at present our philosophy is to treat these women with low-dose aspirin, monitor their LA level during pregnancy and to observe closely as above (Fig. 2.6).

High-titre antibodies (aCL > 60 GPL; KCT > 250 s). Patients in this group require active treatment, with close monitoring of the mother and fetus. The controlled trial published recently by Cowchock et al (1992) found no significant difference in terms of outcome between those treated with heparin and aspirin versus prednisone and aspirin. The policy at present in this institution is to treat those women with previous thrombotic events, particularly deep venous thrombosis, with heparin 10 000 IU b.d. With the

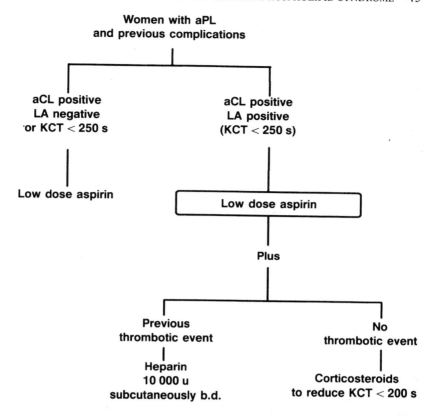

Fig. 2.6 Management plan for women with aPL and previous pregnancy complications.

remaining patients we discuss the treatment options and side-effects and allow the patient to choose (Fig. 2.6).

Patients with previous thrombotic events. All these women are treated with heparin 10 000 IU subcutaneously twice daily.

Drugs available

Aspirin

Aspirin in low dose (75 mg per day) is used extensively. The results of the CLASP trial hopefully will confirm the safety of this medication. Aspirin in low doses does have adverse haemostatic effects — a prolongation of bleeding time occurs — but the incidence of clinically significant bleeding episodes is extremely low.

Heparin

Heparin has considerable side-effects and is of major inconvenience to the patient. A dosage of 10 000 IU twice daily is used in women with previous thromboembolism or those with aPL in high titre. Heparin complications include osteoporosis, thrombocytopenia and bleeding.

Corticosteroids

Although they are frequently used there remain no placebo-controlled trials to demonstrate efficacy of this treatment. Nor has dosage been addressed by trial design. Steroid use is associated with weight gain, acne, hypertension, diabetes and proteinuria. The steroid dose is titrated against the KCT value to maintain a KCT value below 200 s, usually commencing with prednisone 40 mg and measuring KCT values monthly. Frequently a low dose of prednisone (10–20 mg daily) will be sufficient for maintenance. Administration of corticosteroids will suppress the LA but not aCL.

SUMMARY AND FUTURE DIRECTIONS

Antiphospholipid antibodies are described in a wide variety of medical and obstetric disorders. APS is often although not invariably associated with an adverse obstetric outcome. The exact prospective risk of pregnancy loss in women with aPL and prior pregnancy loss is unknown but may exceed 60%.

The mechanism of action of these antibodies remains elusive. A decidual vasculopathy is frequently observed and this would suggest an effect on the vascular endothelium. The central role of the endothelium in normal haemostasis would make this a logical explanation. However, no single abnormality of haemostatic function can be consistently demonstrated in individuals with aPL; this possibly reflects the heterogeneous nature of these antibodies.

The diverse range of tests available for the detection of aPL compounds the literature on aPL. The lack of an internationally standardized unit for reporting and the range of cut-off levels used for positivity of aCL further complicate the issue. Until these basic issues are standardized interpretation of the plethora of papers published on aPL will remain difficult.

Antiphospholipid antibodies are found in 2–3% of the general obstetric population and, owing to low specificity of the tests, mass screening at present does not seem justified. In women with pregnancies complicated by prior fetal losses, abruption, growth retardation or severe early-onset pre-eclampsia, it is prudent to test for these antibodies. Once identified these pregnancies should be regarded as high risk, with referral to a tertiary centre where perinatal, haematological and neonatal expertise is available. Close antenatal supervision of both mother and her fetus should be instituted with careful assessment for maternal thrombotic events, gestational hypertension or fetal growth retardation. There is no clear answer when pharmacological intervention is necessary and, if so, which drugs to use. In the literature to date there is only one randomized controlled trial which compares corticosteroids plus aspirin with heparin and aspirin. No difference in livebirth rate was found, although the steroid group had a higher incidence of premature rupture of membranes. This study contained only 20 subjects and lacked a placebo arm. There is an urgent need for large multicentre trials to address the question of treatment options in pregnancies complicated by the presence of aPL.

There is a need for more scientific research to be performed looking at how these antibodies cause their observed effects, so that more appropriate treatment strategies can be designed. The questions about management of a pregnancy complicated by aPL do not end, however, with the delivery of the baby. The long-term prognosis of the mother remains unknown, and whether long-term pharmacological treatment is indicated to prevent thrombosis is also unclear.

REFERENCES

Andersson L O (1979) Physiochemical properties of antithrombin III. In: Collen D, Wiman B, Verstraete M (eds) The physiological inhibitors of coagulation and fibrinolysis. Elsevier/North-Holland Biomedical Press, Amsterdam, pp 39–42

Asherson R A, Baguley E, Pal C, Hughes G R V 1991 Antiphospholipid syndrome: five year follow-up. Ann Rheum Dis 50: 805–810

Barbui T, Cortelazzo S, Galli M et al 1988 Antiphospholipid antibodies in early repeated abortions: a case controlled study. Fertil Steril 50: 589–592

Birdsall M A, Pattison N S, Chamley L W 1992 Antiphospholipid antibodies in pregnancy. Aust NZ J Obstet Gynaecol 32: 328–330

Blumenfeld Z et al 1991 Anticardiolipin antibodies in patients with recurrent pregnancy wastage: treatment and uterine blood flow. Obstet Gynecol 78: 584–589

Branch W D 1991 Antiphospholipid syndrome: laboratory concerns, fetal loss and pregnancy management. Semin Perinatol 15: 230–237

Branch W D, Scott J R, Kochenour N K et al 1985 Obstetric complications associated with the lupus anticoagulant. N Engl J Med 313: 1322–1326

Branch D W, Andrew R, Digre K B et al 1989 The association of antiphospholipid antibodies with severe pre-eclampsia. Obstet Gynecol 73: 541–545

Branch D W, Rote N S, Dostal D A, Scott J R 1987 Association of lupus anticoagulant with antibody against phosphotidyl serine. Clin Immunol Immunopathol 42: 63–75

Branch D W, Dudley D J, Mitchell M D et al 1990 Immunoglobulin G fractions from patients with antiphospholipid antibodies cause fetal death in BALB/c mice: a model for autoimmune fetal loss. Am J Obstet Gynecol 163: 210–216

Branch D W et al 1990 Antiphospholipid antibody syndrome (APAS): treated pregnancy outcome and medical followup. Proceedings of the 37th Annual Meeting of the Society for Gynecologic Investigation (abstract), p 285.

Brossens I, Robertson W B, Dixon H G 1967 The physiological response of the vessels of the placental bed to normal pregnancy. J Pathol Bacteriol 93: 569–579

Carreras L O, Machin S J, Deman R et al 1981 Arterial thrombosis, intrauterine death and lupus anticoagulant: detection of immunoglobulin interfering with prostacyclin formation. Lancet i: 224–226

Carreras L O, Perez G N, Vega R H, Casavilla F 1988 Lupus anticoagulant and recurrent fetal loss: successful treatment with gamma globulin. Lancet ii: 393–394

Cervera R, Khamashta M A, Font J et al 1991 Antiendothelial cell antibodies in patients with the antiphospholipid syndrome. Autoimmunity 11: 1–6

Chamley L W, McKay E J, Pattison N S 1991a Cofactor depedent and cofactor independent anticardiolipin antibodies. Thromb Res 61: 291–299

Chamley L W, Pattison N S, McKay E J 1991b Separation of lupus anticoagulant from anticardiolipin antibodies by ion-exchange and gel filtration chromatography. Haemostasis 21: 25–29

Chamley L W, McKay E J, Pattison N S 1993 Inhibition of heparin/antithrombin III cofactor activity by anticardiolipin antibodies a mechanism for thrombosis. Thromb Res 71: 103–111

Cines D B, Lyss A P, Reeber M et al 1984 Presence of complement-fixing anti-endothelial cell antibodies in systemic lupus erythematosus. J Clin Invest 73: 611–625

Clauvel J P, Tchobroutsky J C, Danon F et all 1986 Spontaneous recurrent fetal wastage and autoimmune abnormalities: a study of 14 cases. Clin Immunol Immunopathol 39: 523

Comp P C 1990 Laboratory evaluation of protein S status. Semin Thromb Hemost 16: 177–181

Conley L, Hartmann R C 1952 A hemorrhagic disorder caused by circulating anticoagulant in patients with disseminated lupus erythematosus. J Clin Invest 31: 621–622

Cowchock S, Balaban D J 1990 Efficacy of prednisone treatment to prevent recurrent fetal death. Am J Obstet Gynecol 162: 1128

Cowchock F S, Reece E A, Balaban D et al 1992 Repeated fetal losses associated with antiphospholipid antibodies: a collaborative randomised trial comparing prednisone with low dose heparin treatment. Am J Obstet Gynecol 166: 1318–1323

Creagh M D, Greaves M 1991 Lupus anticoagulant. Blood Rev 5: 162–167

Creagh M D, Malia R G, Greaves M 1991 The use of and evacuated collection system in screening for the lupus anticoagulant by the KCCT and DRVVT. Br J Haematol 77: 59

De Wolf F, Carrera L O, Moerman P et al 1982 Decidual vasculopathy and extensive placental infarction in a patient with repeated thromboembolic accidents, recurrent fetal loss and a lupus anticoagulant. Am J Obstet Gynecol 142: 829–834

Exner T, Rickard K, Kronenberg H 1978 A sensitive test demonstrating lupus anticoagulant and its behavioural patterns. Br J Haematol 40: 143–151

Exner T, Sahman N, Trudinger B 1988 Separation of anticardiolipin antibodies from lupus anticoagulant on a phospholipid-coated polystyrene column. Biochem Biophys Res Commun 155: 1001–1007

Farquharson R G et al 1984 Lupus anticoagulant and pregnancy management. Lancet ii: 228

Freyssinet J-M, Wiesel M L, Gauchy J et al 1986 An IgM lupus anticoagulant that neutralises the enhancing effect of phospholipid on purified endothelial thrombomodulin activity: A mechanism for thrombosis. Thromb Haemost 55: 309–313

Galli M, Comfurius P, Maassen C et al 1990a Anticardiolipin antibodies (aCL) directed not to cardiolipin but to a plasma protein cofactor. Lancet 335: 1544–1547

Galli M, Cortelazzo S, Barbui T 1990b Lack of cross-reactivity between anticardiolipin antibodies and glycosaminoglycans. Thromb Res 59: 363–367

Gardlund B 1984 The lupus inhibitor in thromboembolic disease and intrauterine death in the absence of systemic lupus. Acta Med Scand 215: 293

Gatenby P et al 1989 Pregnancy loss with phospholipid antibodies: improved outcome with aspirin containing treatment. Aust NZ J Obstet Gynecol 29: 294–298

Gerrard J M, Friesen L L 1985 Platelets. In: Poller L (ed) Recent advances in blood coagulation, Vol 4. Churchill Livingstone, Edinburgh, pp 139–168

Gregorini G, Setti G, Remuzzi G 1986 Recurrent abortion with lupus anticoagulant and pre-eclampsia: a common final pathology for two different diseases? Br J Obstet Gynaecol 93: 194–196

Hanley J G, Rajaraman S, Behmann S, Denburg J A 1988 A novel neuronal antigen identified by sera from patients with systemic lupus erythematosus. Arthritis Rheum 31: 1492–1499

Harris E N 1987 The syndrome of the black swan. Br J Haematol 26: 324–326

Harris E N 1990 A reassessment of the antiphospholipid antibody syndrome. J Rheumatol 17: 733–735

Harris E N, Spinnato J A 1992 Should cardiolipin tests be performed on otherwise healthy pregnant women? Am J Obstet Gynecol 165: 1272–1277

Harris E N, Gharavi A E, Boey M L et al 1983 Anticardiolipin antibodies: detection by radioimmunoassay and association with thrombosis in systemic lupus erythematosus. Lancet ii: 1211–1214

Harris E N, Gharavi A E, Hedge U et al 1985 Anticardiolipin antibodies in autoimmune thrombocytopaenic purpura. Br J Haematol 59: 231–234

Harris E N, Gharavi A E, Patel S P, Hughes G R V 1987 Evaluation of the anticardiolipin antibody test: report of an international workshop held 4 April 1986. Clin Exp Immunol 68: 215–222

Harris E N, Asherson R A, Hughes G R V 1988 Antiphospholipid antibodies: autoantibodies with a difference. Annu Rev Med 39: 261–271

Hartikalner S, Lilja A. 1980 SLE and habitual abortion. Br J Gynaecol 87: 729–731

Hasselaar P, Derksen R H W M, Blokziji L, De Groot K P G 1988 Thrombosis associated with antiphospholipid antibodies cannot be explained by effects on endothelial and platelet prostanoid synthesis. Thromb Haemost 59: 80–85

Hazeltine M, Rauch J, Danoff D et al 1988 Antiphospholipid antibodies in systemic lupus erythematosus: evidence of an association with positive Coombs and hypocomplementemia. J Rheumatol 15: 80–86

Hecht E R 1965 Lipids in blood clotting. Charles C Thomas, Springfield, IL

Hedfors E, Lindahl G, Lindblad S 1987 Anticardiolipin antibodies during pregnancy. J Rheumatol 14: 160–161

Helgren M, Tengburn L, Abidgard U 1982 Pregnancy in women with congenital antithrombin III deficiency. Gynaecol Obstet Invest 14: 127–141

Infante-Rivard C, David M, Gauthier R, Rivard G E 1991 Lupus anticoagulants, anticardiolipin antibodies and fetal loss. N Engl J Med 325: 1063–1066

Khamashta M A, Harris E N, Gharavi A E et al 1988 Immune mediated mechanism for thrombosis: antiphospholipid antibody binding to platelet membranes. Ann Rheum Dis 47: 849–854

Kwaan H C 1989 Protein C and protein S. Semin Thromb Hemost 15: 353–355

Lesperance B, David M, Rauch J et al 1988 Relative sensitivity of different tests in the dection of low titre lupus anticoagulants. Thromb Haemost 60: 217–219

Lockshin M D, Druzin M L, Goein S et al 1985 Antibody to cardiolipin as a predictor of fetal distress of death in pregnancy patients with systemic lupus erythematosus. N Engl J Med 313: 152

Lockshin M D, Druzin M L, Qamar T 1989 Prednisone does not prevent recurrent fetal death in women with antiphospholipid antibody. Am J Obstet Gynecol 160: 439–443

Lockshin M D, Quamar T, Druzin M, Goei S 1987 Antibody to cardiolipn, lupus anticoagulant and fetal death. J Rheumatol 14: 259–262

Lockwood C J, Romero R, Fienberg R F et al 1989 The prevalence and biologic significance of lupus anticoagulant and anticardiolipin antibodies in a general obstetric population. Am J Obstet Gynecol 161: 369–373

Love P E, Santoro S A 1990 Antiphospholipid antibodies: anticardiolipin and the lupus anticoagulant in systemic lupus erythematosus (SLE) and in non-SLE disorders. Ann Intern Med 112: 682–698

Lubbe W F, Pattison N S 1991 Antiphospholipid antibody syndrome and recurrent fetal loss. Curr Obstet Gynaecol 1: 196–202

Lubbe W F, Palmer S J, Butler W S, Liggins G C 1983 Fetal survival after prednisone suppression of maternal lupus anticoagulant. Lancet i: 1361–1363

Machin S J, Giddings J, Greaves M et al 1990 Detection of lupus-like anticoagulant: current laboratory practice in the United Kingdom. J Clin Pathol 43: 73–75

Marcum J A, Reilly C F, Rosenberg R D 1986 The role of specific forms of heparan sulphate in regulating blood vessel wall function. Prog Hemost Throm 8: 185–215

Masala C, Sorice M, Di Prima M A et al 1989 Evidence for shared epitopes between cardiolipin and *Pneumocystis carinii*. Infect Dis 160: 736–737

Matsuura E, Igarashi Y, Fujimoto M et al 1990 Anticardiolipin cofactor(s) and differential diagnosis of autoimmune disease. Lancet 336: 177–178

McNeil H P, Krilis S A, Chesterman C N 1988 Purification of antiphospholipid antibodies using a new affinity method. Thromb Res 52: 641–648

McNeil H P, Simpson R J, Chesterman C N, Krilis S A 1990 Antiphospholipid antibodies are directed against a complex antigen that includes a lipid-binding inhibitor of coagulation: β_2 glycoprotein 1 (apolipoprotein H). Proc Natl Acad Sci USA 87: 4120–4124

Nilsson I M, Astedt B, Hedner U et al 1975 Intrauterine death and circulating anticoagulant ('antithromboplastin'). Acta Med Scand 197: 153–159

Nimpf J, Wurm H, Kostner G M 1987 B_2 glycoprotein 1 (apo-H) inhibits the release reaction of human platelets during ADP-induced aggregation. Atherosclerosis 63: 109–114

Norberg R, Nived O, Sturfelt G et al 1987 Anticardiolipin and complement activation: relation to clinical symptoms. J Rheumatol 14: 149

Ordi J, Barqueinero J, Vilardell M et al 1989 Fetal loss treatment in patients with antiphospholipid antibodies. Ann Rheum Dis 48: 798–802

Parazzini F, Ackia D, Faden D et al 1991 Antiphospholipid antibodies and recurrent abortion. Obstet Gynecol 77: 854

Parke A L, Wilson D, Bayer-Maierd 1991 The prevalence of antiphospholipid antibodies in women with recurrent spontaneous abortion, women with successful pregnancies and women who have never been pregnant. Arthritis Rheum 34: 1231–1235

Pattison N S, McKay E J, Liggins G C, Lubbe W E 1987 Anticardiolipin antibodies: their presence as a marker for lupus anticoagulant in pregnancy. NZ Med J 100: 61–64

Pattison N S, Chamley L W, McKay E J et al 1993 Antiphospholipid antibodies in pregnancy: prevalence and clinical associations. Br J Obstet Gynaecol 100 (in press)

Peaceman A M, Silver R K, MacGregor S N, Socol M L 1992 Interlaboratory variation in antiphospholipid antibodies testing. Am J Obstet Gynecol 166: 1780–1787

Pengo V, Thiagarajan P, Shapiro S S, Heine M J 1987 Immunological specificity and mechanism of action of IgG lupus anticoagulants. Blood 70: 69–76

Perez M C, Wilson W A, Brown H L, Scopelitise E 1991 Anticardiolipin antibodies in unselected pregnant women in relationship to fetal outcome. J Perinatol 11: 33–36

Reece E A, Gabrielle S, Cullen M T et al 1990 Recurrent adverse pregnancy outcome and antiphospholipid antibodies. Am J Obstet Gynecol 163: 162–169

Ros J, Tarres M V, Raucello M V et al 1983 Prednisone and maternal lupus anticoagulant. Lancet i: 576

Rosove M H et al 1990 Heparin therapy for women with LA or aCL. Obstet Gynecol 75: 630

Rustin M H A, Bull H A, Machin S J et al 1988 Effects of the lupus anticoagulant in patients with systemic lupus erythematosus on endothelial cell prostacyclin release and procoagulant activity. J Invest Dermatol 90: 744–748

Schorer A E, Whickham N W R, Watson K V 1989 Lupus anticoagulant induces a selective defect in thrombin-mediated endothelial prostacyclin release and platelet aggregation. Br J Haematol 71: 399–407

Schousboe I 1985 B_2 glycoprotein 1: a plasma inhibitor of the contact activation of the intrinsic blood coagulation pathway. Blood 66: 1086–1091

Schulman L E 1987 Systemic lupus erythematosus and the chronic biologic false positive test of syphilis. In: Wallace D J, Dubois E L (eds) Dubois' lupus erythematosus, 3rd Edn. Lea & Febiger, Philadelphia

Schulze-Lohoft E, Krapf F, Bleil L et al 1989 IgM-containing immune complexes and antiphospholipid antibodies in patients with Snedden's syndrome. Rheum Int 9: 43–48

Scott Jr et al 1988 Intravenous immunoglobulin treatment of pregnant patients with recurrent pregnancy loss caused by antiphospholipid antibodies and Rh immunisation. Am J Obstet Gynecol 159: 1055

Shapiro S, Thiagarajan P 1982 Lupus anticoagulants. Prog Hemost Thromb 6: 263–285

Shi W, Krilis S A, Chong B H et al 1990 Prevalence of lupus anticoagulant and anticardiolipin antibodies in a healthy population. Aust NZ J Med 20: 231–236

Toyoshima K, Makino, Suji T et al 1991 Correlation between trimester of fetal wastage and anticardiolipin antibody titre. Int J Fertil 32: 89–93

Triplett D A, Brandt J T 1989 Laboratory identification of the lupus anticoagulant. Br J Haematol 73: 139–142

Tsakiris D A, Settas L, Makris P E, Marbet G A 1990 Lupus anticoagulant, antiphospholipid antibodies and thrombophilia: relation to protein C-protein S-thrombomodulin. J Rheumatol 17: 785–789

Unander A M, Norbert R, Hahn L, Arfors L 1987 Anticardiolipin antibodies and complement in ninety-nine women with habitual abortion. Am J Obstet Gynecol 156: 114–119

Wurm H 1984 B_2 glycoprotein 1 (apolipoprotein H) interactions with phospholipid vesicles. Int J Biochem 16: 511–515

3

Advances in the management of diabetes in pregnancy: success through simplicity

M. D. G. Gillmer   N. J. Bickerton

HISTORICAL PERSPECTIVE

In 1824 Bennewitz, published the first case report of gestational diabetes. This formed the basis of his MD thesis 'Diabetes Mellitus: A Symptom of Pregnancy'. In addition to the classic diabetic symptoms and signs of thirst, polyuria and associated glycosuria, he described the death of a macrosomic fetus due to impacted shoulders (cited in Hadden 1989). The patient's diabetes resolved completely after delivery, but recurred in two subsequent pregnancies. Many years later in 1882, J. Matthews Duncan read a paper before the London Obstetrical Society in which he reported the outcome of 22 pregnancies in 15 women. The fetal loss was 47%. Four of the women died in coma or collapse after delivery, and 7 others died within 2 years of the pregnancy — a maternal mortality of 73%. The most comprehensive review of diabetes in pregnancy in the pre-insulin era was, however, published in 1909 by J. Whitridge Williams, of the Johns Hopkins University in Baltimore. He was careful to distinguish between physiological glycosuria and true diabetes, and presented a review of 57 pregnancies between 1874 and 1909 involving 34 women. The maternal mortality in this series was 25% and only 51% of women gave birth to a living child.

Insulin became generally available in 1923 and the first major appraisal of its effects in pregnancy complicated by diabetes was published by Skipper from the London Hospital in 1933. He presented information on 136 pregnancies in 118 women collected from the world literature and also a personal series of 36 pregnancies in 33 women. He observed that although maternal mortality had fallen dramatically with insulin treatment to 9.6% in the review series and 3% in his personal series, the fetal mortality in the two series remained very high at 45.2% and 40.5%, respectively. These and other historical reviews form the backdrop against which the effectiveness of modern management can be judged and will be referred to in this chapter to demonstrate that the outcome that can be achieved nowadays in diabetic pregnancies is due as much to modern technology as to our enhanced understanding of the pathology of diabetes in pregnancy.

A recent Medline search revealed that during the last 25 years more than 4000 papers on diabetes in pregnancy have been published in the English language alone. To perform a comprehensive review of the literature on the subject would therefore be impossible. This chapter therefore represents a personal view of the modern management of diabetes in pregnancy, with a highly selective review of the literature.

GESTATIONAL DIABETES

... the diabetes appeared in the patient along with the pregnancy and at the very same time; when the pregnancy appeared it appeared; while pregnancy lasted it lasted; as pregnancy developed it developed; and it terminated soon after the pregnancy. (H. G. Bennewitz 1824)

This statement, made nearly 170 years ago, is undoubtedly the earliest description of gestational diabetes. This condition is now recognized to be due to the progressive insulin resistance that develops during pregnancy as a consequence of the secretion of placental hormones into the maternal circulation, in particular progesterone and human placental lactogen (hPL). The current widely accepted definition of gestational diabetes agreed at the Second International Workshop Conference on Gestational Diabetes (Proceedings 1985) is 'carbohydrate intolerance of variable severity with onset or first recognition during the present pregnancy'. This rather loose definition was coupled with the glucose tolerance criteria for the diagnosis of gestational diabetes established by O'Sullivan and Mahan in 1964 using a 100 g oral glucose load. Although these diagnostic criteria have been accepted by the American Diabetes Association (ADA) and the American College of Obstetricians and Gynecologists (ACOG) for the diagnosis of gestational diabetes in North America, the 75 g oral glucose tolerance test (GTT) has been widely accepted elsewhere, especially in Europe. The criteria for diagnosing gestational diabetes, regardless of the size of the glucose load, have, however, proved to be controversial.

The WHO (1980) recommended that the criteria for 'impaired glucose tolerance' in the non-pregnant should be used to diagnose 'gestational diabetes'. This rather simplistic approach, however, ignores not only the physiological changes in glucose tolerance that occur during pregnancy but also the fact that the study population for the WHO criteria did not include any pregnant women! The result is that when the WHO criteria are applied to a pregnant population the incidence of 'gestational diabetes' is unrealistically high. Indeed, a study of the 75 g oral GTT in 491 women at 28–32 weeks gestation performed in Oxford revealed that 14.4% of women had a 2-hour plasma glucose in excess of 8.0 mmol/l (Table 3.1).

Despite this there was no demonstrable adverse outcome in these pregnancies and we have therefore adopted the figure of 9.5 mmol/l (mean plus two standard deviations) as the upper limit of normal for the 75 g oral GTT in the third trimester of pregnancy. This figure is in broad agreement with others (Table 3.2) including the findings of the Diabetic Pregnancy Study Group (DPSG) of the European Association of the Study for Diabetes

Table 3.1 Incidence of 'impaired glucose tolerance' (gestational diabetes) and 'Diabetes' by WHO criteria in the Oxford Study

2-hour plasma glucose	No. of patients (n = 486)	Percentage
<8 mmol/l	416	85.6
8–11 mmol/l	65	13.4
>11 mmol/l	5	1.0

Table 3.2 Upper limits for normal oral glucose tolerance criteria[a] in pregnancy

	DPSG/EASD (75 g)	Oxford (75 g)	WHO (75 g)	ADA/ACOG (100 g)
Fasting	5.4	6.0	< 8	5.8
1-hour	11.1	12.5		10.5
2-hour	9.1	9.5	8–11	9.2
3-hour	8.3	7.5		8.1

[a]Venous plasma glucose (mmol/l).

(EASD) (Lind & Phillips 1991) and with the figure derived from O'Sullivan & Mahan (1964) for a 100 g oral GTT.

SCREENING FOR GESTATIONAL DIABETES

I know of no complication of pregnancy the significance of which is more variously interpreted than the presence of sugar in the urine of pregnant women. Certain writers regard it as a harmless almost physiological phenomenon, while others hold that it is always indicative of diabetes. (J. Whitridge Williams 1909)

More than 80 years after this statement was made the benefit of testing urine for glucose and the role of glycosuria in screening for gestational diabetes remain uncertain. Indeed the whole question of screening for gestational diabetes is extremely controversial. Although only very few units have abandoned routine antenatal testing for glycosuria, many now rely on blood glucose measurements for the detection of gestational diabetes. The most strict protocol for screening is that advocated by the Second International Workshop Conference on Gestational Diabetes in 1985, which recommended that 'All pregnant women should be screened for glucose intolerance' and that they should receive 'a glucose load between the 24th and 28th wk consisting of 50 g oral glucose given without regard to the time of the last meal or the time of day'. Venous plasma glucose is measured an hour later, and a value equal to or greater than 140 mg/dl (7.8 mmol/l) is recommended as the threshold for a full diagnostic GTT. This system originally validated by O'Sullivan and co-workers in Boston (1973) is undoubtedly the most sensitive (79%) and specific (87%) means of identifying abnormal glucose tolerance in pregnancy. Considerable geographical variation in the incidence of gestational diabetes exists and such a costly and inconvenient system may not be justified in populations with a low prevalence of diabetes mellitus. An alternative screening system based on random antenatal plasma glucose estimations in the early third trimester has been proposed by Lind (1985) and has achieved some popularity, especially in Europe. Although much more convenient than techniques involving glucose loading it appears to be a great deal less sensitive and specific. Measurement of glycosylated proteins such as haemoglobin (HbA₁C) or plasma protein and fructosamine assays have seemed attractive because of their relative simplicity, but in practice have proved to be too insensitive for routine screening for gestational diabetes (Roberts et al 1990).

'Should all pregnant women be screened for gestational glucose intolerance?' This question was posed by Ales & Santini (1989) in an excellent overview of the subject. They concluded that despite the wide acceptance of blood-based screening programmes there is no evidence to suggest that gestational glucose intolerance is associated with excess fetal mortality, or maternal or fetal morbidity. There does, however, appear to be evidence that gestational glucose intolerance is associated with an excess of heavy infants and some evidence that this can be reduced by treatment with insulin (Coustan 1991). Women identified as gestational diabetics are at increased risk of developing maturity-onset diabetes, and avoidance of obesity in middle age may prevent the development of diabetes in these women (O'Sullivan 1991). Ales & Santini (1989) concluded that 'The scientific data supporting a universal screening programme for gestational glucose intolerance showing that treatment of gestational diabetes does more good than harm are limited' and that until this is available 'a more restrained approach than universal screening might be appropriate'. Pregnancy induces decompensated diabetes in a number of women, and the incidence of this condition is dependent not only on the underlying prevalence of diabetes in the population (Green et al 1990) but also on the age of the women (McFarland & Case 1985). The intensity of screening for gestational diabetes in any particular population should therefore take into account both the age and ethnic origin of the women screened and should aim to define the severity of glucose intolerance. The 50 g oral glucose challenge is undoubtedly the 'gold standard' by which other techniques must be judged when screening pregnant women in populations with a high prevalence of diabetes mellitus. In those communities with a low prevalence of this condition its use cannot easily be justified because of the cost and inconvenience entailed, and the limited clinical benefit.

Oxford has a relatively low-risk population, and we have aimed to identify those women who develop decompensated diabetes during pregnancy (i.e. those with preprandial plasma glucose measurements consistently in excess of 6 mmol/l when consuming a normal diet). We have combined traditional urine analysis with random blood glucose testing. In practice urine is tested for glycosuria at every clinic visit and, if detected, blood is taken for a 'timed-random' blood glucose measurement. If the plasma glucose is more than 6 mmol/l in the fasting state or 2 hours or more after a meal or snack or more than 7 mmol/l up to 2 hours after a meal or snack then a 75 g oral GTT is performed. If any of the oral GTT criteria listed in Table 3.2 are exceeded then the woman is tested preprandially before each meal or snack, while consuming a normal mixed diet, at the times shown in the Obstetric Diabetic Record (Fig. 3.1).

If this 'preprandial series' reveals plasma glucose concentrations of between 6 and 8 mmol/l, a high-fibre diet is advised, with a reduced caloric content if the woman is eating excessively or is obese. She is then retested while consuming this diet. If the preprandial plasma glucose concentrations initially exceed 8 mmol/l or remain above 6 mmol/l, on an appropriate diet, then insulin therapy is commenced, using a long-acting preparation in the first instance. Preprandial short-acting insulin is added before meals if the postprandial, i.e. pre-snack, values remain above 6 mmol/l. Oral hypo-glycaemics are not used because they cross the placenta and stimulate the fetal pancreatic β-cells, causing fetal hyperinsulinaemia — the pathological process that insulin treatment aims to avoid.

Glycosuria has been deemed too insensitive and non-specific to form the basis of a screening programme for gestational diabetes. This is only true if one aims to detect very minor degrees of glucose intolerance. Our aim has been to identify those women with decompensated diabetes (see above), and in our experience most of them have glycosuria on at least one occasion. In addition, Pettitt et al (1980) have demonstrated that 74% of Pima women with a blood glucose concentration of 11 mM or more 2 hours after a 75 g oral glucose load, administered in the third trimester, had glycosuria. The Oxford screening protocol was also assessed by means of a retrospective review of perinatal deaths in 18 811 deliveries at the John Radcliffe Hospital between January 1978 and June 1981. During this period there were 121 first-week neonatal deaths and 75 stillbirths. The postmortem reports were scrutinized for evidence of undiagnosed diabetes as the cause of the perinatal death, in particular evidence of fetal pancreatic β-cell hyperplasia. Ten perinatal deaths were in babies whose birthweight exceeded the 90th centile; only one of these was designated as an 'unexplained' stillbirth. Of the remaining 9, 5 were due to congenital abnormalities, 3 to intrapartum asphyxia, and 1 was a 'cot death'. The *potentially* avoidable perinatal mortality due to possible undiag-nosed diabetes was therefore 0.05 per 1000. In the absence of fetal pancreatic β-cell hyperplasia this seems an unlikely cause of this single death.

MEDICAL MANAGEMENT OF DIABETES IN PREGNANCY

During treatment, constant supervision and rigid control of the blood-sugar are of great importance. Only thus can a living child be obtained with reasonable certainty. (E. Skipper 1933)

Oxfordshire Health Authority   **John Radcliffe Maternity Hospital**

OBSTETRIC   DIABETIC   RECORD

Patient details:					Month:	Year:	Key to Test-time codes: PB: pre-b'fast
					Insulin(s): A: B:		PC: pre-coffee PL: pre-lunch PT: pre-tea PS: pre-supper BT: bed-time

Date	Time of test	Blood glucose	Insulin dose A	B	Sign here	Comments	Hypos (time)	Urine glucose	Ketones
Sunday	PB								
	PC								
	PL								
	PT								
	PS								
	BT								
Monday	PB								
	PC								
	PL								
	PT								
	PS								
	BT								
Tuesday	PB								
	PC								
	PL								
	PT								
	PS								
	BT								
Wednesday	PB								
	PC								
	PL								
	PT								
	PS								
	BT								
Thursday	PB								
	PC								
	PL								
	PT								
	PS								
	BT								
Friday	PB								
	PC								
	PL								
	PT								
	PS								
	BT								
Saturday	PB								
	PC								
	PL								
	PT								
	PS								
	BT								

OH 2544

Fig. 3.1   The obstetric diabetic record form.

Despite reporting a fetal mortality of 45.2% in a collected series of 136 pregnancies and of 40.5% in a personal series of 37 pregnancies, Skipper was able, only a decade after the introduction of insulin, to recognize that 'rigid' control of diabetes during pregnancy was essential for a successful outcome, and observed that 'By far the most important cause of foetal death is neglect of the diabetes, especially during the latter months of pregnancy'. It was not until 50 years later, however, that perinatal mortality rates consistently below 10% were achieved; results comparable to those of non-diabetic women have only been obtained in the last decade. Gabbe (1980), in his masterly review entitled 'Management of Diabetes in Pregnancy: Six Decades of Experience', traced the history of the management of this condition and identified four distinct periods: 1921–1940, which he described as the period of maternal insulin therapy; 1941–1970, designated as the period of team care; 1971–1976, the period of fetal surveillance; and 1976 to the present, the period of metabolic normalization (Table 3.3).

Since the mid-1970s two major factors have enabled the greatly improved outcome of diabetic pregnancy. The first was the recognition by Karlsson & Kjellmer (1972) that perinatal mortality in pregnancies complicated by diabetes is directly related to the degree of glycaemic control, especially during the last trimester. In addition, it was recognized that to achieve normoglycaemia preprandial blood glucose concentrations must be reduced to values consistently between 4 and 6 mmol/l. This may be impossible in the majority of type 1 diabetics but nonetheless remains the ultimate goal. Initially this could only be achieved with inpatient management and prolonged hospitalization of all insulin-treated pregnant diabetic women, usually from early in the third trimester of pregnancy until delivery. The second major advance was the development of portable glucose meters that could be used by patients at home. These have been widely available since the late 1970s and have revolutionized patient care. The admission of patients during pregnancy is rarely required unless they are being taught to use insulin for the first time or a serious medical or obstetric problem arises.

Pre-pregnancy care

Diabetes preceding pregnancy is associated with a three- to five-fold increase in the incidence of neural tube, cardiac and renal anomalies, and although

Table 3.3   The evolution of care in diabetic pregnancy

Period	Aim of care	Perinatal mortality (%)	Ratio of stillbirths to neonatal deaths
1921–1940	Avoid ketoacidosis	33.3–29.1	2.0
1941–1970	Team care/early delivery	29.1–18.1	1.3
1971–1976	Fetal surveillance	18.1–12.0	1.6
1976–1992	Aim for normoglycaemia	12.6–<1.0	0.8

this was a relatively unimportant cause of perinatal mortality in the early post-insulin era, the gradual reduction in deaths due to ketoacidosis, trauma, prematurity and late intrauterine deaths means that more than a half of current perinatal deaths are now caused by lethal congenital anomalies. They are also an important cause of long-term morbidity in the offspring of diabetic women. Although the need for special prepregnancy diabetic clinics to prevent congenital malformations has recently been questioned, there can be no doubt that optimal control prior to conception significantly reduces the incidence of these anomalies. Clearly general practitioners, diabetic physicians and specialist diabetic nurses all have an important part to play in educating women about these risks and the need to achieve optimal diabetic control before pregnancy in order to avoid them (Gregory & Tattersall 1992). Given the increased incidence of neural tube defects, folic acid supplementation should be recommended.

Team care

The concept of 'team care' of diabetes in pregnancy first developed in the 1930s and 1940s but is just as important today. The composition of the team has, however, altered subtly in recent years and it cannot be emphasized too strongly that the most important member of this team is *the patient herself*. She, of course has responsibility for her diabetes on a day-to-day basis and usually has the clearest understanding of how *she* can achieve optimal glycaemic control. The other important members of the team include specialist midwives and nurses, a dietitian, and an obstetrician or perinatalologist with a special interest in this problem. Diabetes is usually relatively easy to control during pregnancy because of the progressive increase in insulin resistance and tolerance of hypoglycaemia that develop, together with the very high degree of motivation and compliance shown by most patients. In many hospitals care is often shared with a physician. This is not essential, provided that the obstetrician concerned has been trained in the management of diabetes and has ready access to the advice of a specialist diabetic physician should this be required. Preferably the patient should attend only one clinic at each visit and not have to see the diabetic physician and obstetrician in two different clinics on the same day.

Antenatal visits

Close supervision and constant support are essential during pregnancy, and all diabetics should be seen in the antenatal clinic as early as possible. Thereafter the frequency of clinic visits will depend not only on the degree of control achieved, but also on the occurrence of diabetic or obstetric complications. All diabetic women should be seen at least every 2 weeks until 34 weeks gestation and then weekly until delivery. This facilitates the frequent alterations of insulin dose as the pregnancy progresses and also ensures adequate dietary advice. If control is relatively poor and more frequent advice is required, this can easily be achieved by telephone contact. This avoids the need to admit the patient, which is disruptive to both her pattern of activity and her diet—both important components of her overall diabetic control.

Insulin therapy

Human insulin is preferred, as this produces the lowest antibody concentrations and reduces the theoretical risks of fetal β-cell damage or macrosomia due to the transplacental passage of injected insulin bound to antibody (Menon et al 1990). Despite considerable controversy, there appears to be little evidence to support current concerns that human insulin lessens awareness of hypoglycaemia (Maran et al 1993).

No perfect insulin regime exists for all patients, and in practice the patient's prepregnancy insulin regime should only be changed if it proves impossible to achieve the desired standard of control. The traditional twice-daily use of short and intermediate-acting insulins remains popular, but a variety of new insulin regimes has been introduced in recent years. The continuous subcutaneous insulin infusion (CSII) pump, popularized in the early 1980s, was initially hailed as the ideal means of achieving normoglycaemia. This utilizes a constant basal infusion with premeal boluses as required. Careful studies in both pregnant and non-pregnant subjects have, however, failed to identify any significant advantage over conventional intermittent injections. In addition, the pregnant diabetic is particularly prone to overnight ketoacidosis, and the absence of any insulin depot in women using this system means that disruption of the infusion through pump failure, catheter blockage or disconnection can rapidly lead to ketoacidotic coma, with the risk of fetal or even maternal death. Much of the flexibility of CSII has, however, been retained by combining a single daily injection of long or intermediate-acting insulin, usually administered at bedtime, with three or occasionally more intermittent preprandial injections of short-acting insulin, administered with an insulin 'pen'. Although severe hypoglycaemia is rare during pregnancy, a glucagon 'kit' is given to all pregnant diabetic women at their first antenatal visit as a precaution.

Monitoring glycaemic control

The aim of therapy is to maintain all pre- and postprandial blood glucose measurements between 4 and 6 mmol/l. Insulin dose and blood glucose measurements are recorded on an obstetric diabetic record (see Fig. 3.1). Monitoring blood glucose concentrations using test strips has now become standard practice in all insulin-dependent diabetics. Many non-pregnant patients rely on visual inspection of the colour change of the test strip but this is not acceptable in pregnant women. Glucose meters, which are now extremely cheap, provide a much more accurate indication of blood glucose

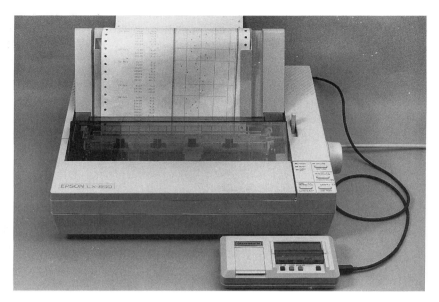

Fig. 3.2 The Ames memory meter and 'intelligent' printer.

and avoid subjective bias. Since 1986 a 'memory meter' (Ames Glucometer-M) with the capacity to store more than 300 glucose concentrations together with the date and time of the measurements has been used by most women attending the Oxford Diabetic Antenatal Clinic. These meters have the advantage that they can be connected to a printer (Fig. 3.2) containing a dedicated microprocessor which calculates the mean blood glucose measurements over the preceding fortnight, a breakdown of all glucose values in the form of a histogram, and a summation of all values in a 'modal day' (see printouts 1–4 in Appendix, pp 75–78).

This protocol for outpatient monitoring of diabetic control using blood glucose meters is extremely cost-effective. The need for admission to hospital is avoided and a much more sensitive indication of short and medium-term glycaemic control is provided than can be achieved with relatively costly and insensitive measurements of glycosylated haemoglobin (HbA_1C).

Retinal assessment

Rapid improvement in the blood glucose concentrations of patients who have previously had poor control may cause deterioration of pre-existing retinopathy (Hare 1991). All women are therefore referred for a full ophthalmic assessment in early pregnancy to determine the need for subsequent supervision or laser therapy.

Management of diabetes during and after labour

Although the need for glucose and insulin infusions in labour has recently been questioned (Yudkin & Knopfler 1992), it is vital to maintain euglycaemia at this time in order to minimize the risk of neonatal hypoglycaemia (Soler et al 1978). In Oxford this is achieved using the system shown in Figure 3.3. Ten per cent dextrose BP is infused at a constant rate to provide 10 g of glucose per hour. Blood glucose measurements are made every hour in the patient's other arm while short-acting (neutral) insulin (6 units in 60 ml normal saline BP) is administered by means of an infusion pump at an initial rate of 1 unit (10 ml) per hour. This is doubled or halved as necessary to maintain the blood glucose concentration between 4 to 6 mmol/l. During labour the insulin requirement may fall dramatically, presumably because of the increased glucose demand due to uterine work, and it is frequently necessary to switch the insulin infusion off towards the end of the first stage (Jovanovic & Peterson 1983).

The insulin infusion rate after delivery should be halved as a rapid decline in insulin sensitivity follows separation of the placenta. It is also essential to return to the prepregnancy insulin dose, immediately the patient resumes her normal diet; profound hypoglycaemia may occur if the dose required prior to delivery is administered.

OBSTETRIC MANAGEMENT OF DIABETES IN PREGNANCY

Within recent years, several authors have advocated caesarean section before term to prevent death in utero. They advise, when the fetus is sufficiently large, to deliver it by section. Such advice is open to question... It is my opinion that the diabetic patient should be delivered per vagina. If the baby is large and it appears that delivery will be difficult, then caesarean section should be resorted to. (M. M. Shir, read at a meeting of the Brooklyn Gynecological Society, 4 November 1938)

Antenatal assessment of the fetus

Accurate information about the duration of pregnancy, fetal growth and fetal well-being remains as important in the management of the pregnant diabetic now as it was when Shir made this statement more than 50 years ago. Since then the use of diagnostic ultrasound has revolutionized our ability to assess the fetus in ways that Shir and his contemporaries could never have dreamed of. Indeed, ultrasound imaging systems have become absolutely central to the modern obstetric management of diabetes in pregnancy, and almost every known use for obstetric ultrasound has a place in the care of the pregnant diabetic.

The first use of ultrasound in diabetic pregnancy is to measure the crown–rump length (CRL) to confirm the duration of pregnancy. This technique, although generally accepted as a means of assessing gestational age in non-diabetics, has proved controversial in diabetic pregnancy. Fog-Pedersen & Molsted-Pedersen (1989) have described a condition of 'early growth delay' in some diabetic women in which the fetal CRL is more than

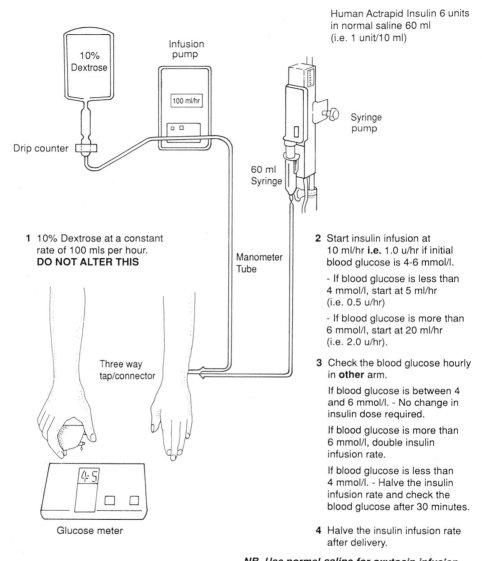

Human Actrapid Insulin 6 units in normal saline 60 ml (i.e. 1 unit/10 ml)

Infusion pump

10% Dextrose

100 ml/hr

Syringe pump

Drip counter

60 ml Syringe

1 10% Dextrose at a constant rate of 100 mls per hour. **DO NOT ALTER THIS**

Manometer Tube

Three way tap/connector

Glucose meter

2 Start insulin infusion at 10 ml/hr **i.e.** 1.0 u/hr if initial blood glucose is 4-6 mmol/l.

- If blood glucose is less than 4 mmol/l, start at 5 ml/hr (i.e. 0.5 u/hr)

- If blood glucose is more than 6 mmol/l, start at 20 ml/hr (i.e. 2.0 u/hr).

3 Check the blood glucose hourly in **other** arm.

If blood glucose is between 4 and 6 mmol/l. - No change in insulin dose required.

If blood glucose is more than 6 mmol/l, double insulin infusion rate.

If blood glucose is less than 4 mmol/l. - Halve the insulin infusion rate and check the blood glucose after 30 minutes.

4 Halve the insulin infusion rate after delivery.

NB. Use normal saline for oxytocin infusion.

Fig. 3.3   Protocol for management of diabetes during labour.

6 days smaller than the gestational age calculated from certain menstrual dates. They have reported that this 'growth delay' is associated with an increased rate of congenital malformations and poor fetal growth (Table 3.4).

Table 3.4 Incidence of severe congenital malformations related to fetal size, expressed as the difference between the gestational age (calculated from the last menstrual period in women with certain dates) and the gestational age calculated from a CRL measurement in the first trimester of pregnancy

Gestational age difference	Incidence of severe congenital malformations
Less then 6 days too small	3/131 (2%)
More than 6 days too small	10/70 (14%)

These authors have suggested that early growth delay is a result of 'less than optimal' metabolic compensation in early pregnancy. If this is confirmed it will serve to emphasize the importance of achieving normoglycaemia before conception and during the first trimester of pregnancy.

A biparietal diameter measurement should also be performed in the mid-trimester, ideally at 16 weeks gestation, to provide additional information about gestational age. Blood for serum α-fetoprotein can also be taken at this gestation both to screen for neural tube defects and as part of the 'triple test' used to screen for Down's syndrome. Wald et al (1992) have demonstrated that the serum α-fetoprotein and unconjugated oestriol concentrations observed in diabetic pregnancy are lower than those in non-diabetic women, and this could lead to an erroneous interpretation of these screening tests.

A detailed fetal examination to exclude congenital anomalies especially of the neural, cardiac and renal systems should be performed between 18 and 20 weeks, so that termination of the pregnancy can be considered, if appropriate.

Serial studies of growth based on measurements of the fetal head and abdominal circumferences provide the best means of identifying those pregnancies in which the fetus is becoming macrosomic. Fog-Pedersen & Molsted-Pedersen (1989) have found that the most sensitive indicator of macrosomia in late pregnancy is an abdominal circumference measurement at 28–29 weeks gestation. If this is 1 cm or more above the mean value at this stage of pregnancy then there is a 77% likelihood of fetal macrosomia. This observation highlights two important practical points. First, as the pancreatic β-cells of the fetus of the diabetic appear to become sensitized to circulating insulin secretagogues during the second trimester, as much care should be taken to maintain optimal metabolic control during mid-pregnancy as during the first and third trimesters. In addition, although relative fetal hyperinsulinaemia only has a minor impact on fetal growth at this gestation, it appears to have a much greater impact in later pregnancy. Second, it may be possible to predict macrosomia at a time in pregnancy when it is still possible to institute optimal metabolic control and thus reduce the likelihood of this complication. Special attention should therefore be given to these women to ensure euglycaemia during the third trimester. It should, however, be emphasized that while many studies have demonstrated an association between birthweight and maternal blood glucose concentrations during the third trimester of pregnancy, the cause of macrosomia in the infant of the diabetic woman is not completely clear, and some women can deliver infants with birthweights above the 97th centile despite excellent metabolic control in late pregnancy. On the other hand, Langer and co-workers (1989) have shown a clear relationship between neonatal size (expressed as a birth percentile) and the level of glycaemic control. He observed a more than twofold increase in large-for-gestational-age infants (defined as a birthweight above the 90th centile) in women with a mean blood glucose exceeding 5.8 mmol/l, and a twofold increase in small-for-dates infants (defined as a birthweight below the 10th centile) in those diabetics with very tight control and a mean blood glucose concentration of less than 4.8 mmol/l. These data are important as they indicate that excessively tight blood glucose control may have a deleterious effect on the growth of the diabetic fetus and possibly also on development.

Obstetric complications of diabetes in pregnancy

Proteinuric hypertension. This occurs approximately twice as often in diabetic compared to non-diabetic women (Garner et al 1990). In Oxford maternal serum urate and creatinine concentrations are measured at every antenatal visit and 24-hour urine protein concentrations from 24 weeks gestation. These provide not only the earliest biochemical evidence of proteinuric pre-eclampsia but also serve to clarify blood pressure changes unmasked by pregnancy which are due to pre-existing essential hypertension.

The reason for the increased incidence of pre-eclampsia in pregnancies complicated by diabetes is unknown. A link with glycaemic control has been established, and the incidence of this complication is reduced with optimal metabolic control of the diabetes.

Polyhydramnios. This has long been recognized as one of the hallmarks of diabetic pregnancy, and indeed may be the presenting feature of gestational diabetes, especially in those rare cases where type 1 (insulin-dependent) diabetes develops coincidentally during pregnancy. The cause of this complication, which has an overall incidence of approximately 15% (Cousins 1987), remains uncertain but it is probably due to an osmotic diuresis induced in the fetus by the feto-maternal hyperglycaemia that occurs in uncontrolled or poorly controlled diabetes. The degree of polyhydramnios generally reduces as the diabetic control improves, but treatment with indomethacin, which reduces fetal urine production, has been advocated when this fails to occur (Moise 1991). This therapy may, however, induce premature closure of the ductus arteriosus (Mohen et al 1992).

Premature labour. This is more frequent in diabetic pregnancy (Lufkin et al 1984, Greene et al 1989) and may in some instances be due to underlying polyhydramnios. Conventional management with intravenous β-sympatho-mimetics and glucocorticoids is, however, potentially hazardous as β-sympathomimetic agents cause hepatic glycogenolysis and insulin resistance. Glucocorticoids have an additive effect, and their concurrent use in diabetic pregnant women may necessitate the administration of very high doses of intravenous insulin (up to 30 units per hour) to maintain normoglycaemia and avoid ketoacidosis. Barnett et al (1980) therefore, advised that this therapy should be avoided whenever possible, even in non-insulin-dependent patients, because of the serious risk of ketoacidosis. A subsequent study by Miodovnik et al (1985) agreed with the need for increased doses of insulin to maintain euglycaemia, but concluded that β-sympathomimetic drugs could safely be used to treat premature labour in patients with insulin-dependent diabetes, provided they were administered in a strictly controlled clinical setting. Alternatives that have been suggested include the calcium channel blocker nifedipine and magnesium sulphate (Barss 1989).

Fetal well-being and maturity

We somehow have to be able to find the patient whose infant is at risk of dying before delivery, at the same time allowing the infant, who is not mature enough to exist in an intrauterine environment, a longer period of gestation. (J. J. Delaney & J. Ptacek 1970)

Intrauterine death in late pregnancy was recognized as a major problem in the management of diabetic pregnancy in the late 1930s and 1940s and led to a policy of early delivery. This, unfortunately, was followed by a high Caesarean section rate for failed induction, resulting in an increase in neonatal morbidity and mortality. In the late 1960s and early 1970s biochemical methods of assessing fetal well-being became popular. These initially involved the measurement of urinary excretion products of placental and feto-placental hormones such as pregnanediol and oestriol, and later monitoring of placental hormone concentrations in blood, including oestriol, oestradiol and human placental lactogen (Gillmer & Beard 1975). These indirect techniques of assessing the fetus were, however, replaced in the late 1970s and early 1980s by the more direct ultrasound-based 'biophysical' procedures involving a real-time ultrasound examination of the fetus combined with a fetal resting cardiotocographic tracing, the so-called 'biophysical profile' (Manning et al 1981, Manning 1990). This technique has revolutionized the late pregnancy management of the pregnant diabetic woman and has more or less obviated the need to admit diabetic women in late pregnancy. It has also enabled diabetic pregnancy to be prolonged to near term or beyond (Johnson et al 1988) and it is now standard practice in Oxford to perform biophysical profile assessments on all diabetic pregnant women weekly, during their antenatal clinic visits, from 36 weeks gestation or more frequently if indicated.

Antenatal Doppler ultrasound assessments have also been used widely in recent years. As with the 'biophysical profile' normal results obtained using this technique have provided the reassurance necessary to prolong uncomplicated diabetic pregnancies beyond term. In keeping with the findings of Landon and co-workers (1989) and Johnstone et al (1992) we have not, however, found any association between Doppler velocity waveforms and indices of diabetic control (unpublished observations). We would, however, agree that measurements of the umbilical artery resistance index may be of value in detecting fetal compromise in diabetic pregnancies complicated by intrauterine growth retardation.

Fetal maturity and timing of delivery

My experience with the fourth case was so tragic, I felt so badly about having lost a baby, which died under observation that the general rule was laid down to deliver all these insulin mothers and sick diabetics by caesarean section as soon as it was felt that the baby was viable. (R. S. Titus, read before the Section of Obstetrics and Gynecology, New York Academy of Medicine, 26 November 1935)

Poorly controlled diabetes is associated with fetal pulmonary and hepatic immaturity which predispose to the neonatal respiratory distress syndrome and jaundice. Fear of 'unexplained' intrauterine death in the last 4 weeks of pregnancy, however, led obstetricians to induce labour as soon as the fetus was considered to be mature enough to survive. In 1969 Spellacy, in a detailed review on the timing of delivery in diabetic pregnancy, pointed out that 'Most authors feel this time to be about thirty seven weeks of gestation'. However, even in the late 1960s some obstetricians still advocated delivery between 35 and 37 weeks despite a high overall perinatal mortality of 20–25% at this stage of pregnancy. In the late 1960s and early 1970s, techniques which involved transabdominal amniocentesis were introduced to assess fetal pulmonary maturity by measuring the lecithin–sphingomyelin ratio and phosphatidyl glycerol concentrations in amniotic fluid. Despite their invasive nature, these techniques were rapidly and enthusiastically accepted by obstetricians as a part of the routine management of the insulin-dependent diabetic not only in an effort to reduce the perinatal morbidity and mortality associated with fetal pulmonary immaturity but also to allow the pregnancy to be prolonged towards term. During the late 1970s it became increasingly apparent that late 'unexplained' stillbirths were largely due to poor diabetic control, and that fetal 'immaturity' and the associated perinatal morbidity and mortality observed before 38 weeks were largely due to Caesarean section, either elective or emergency (Roberts et al 1976) — the latter following fetal distress or failed attempts to induce women with unripe cervices. In women with good diabetic control, pregnancy should, whenever possible, be allowed to progress beyond 38 weeks gestation in order to minimize the complications due to iatrogenic prematurity and improve the likelihood of spontaneous labour and a vaginal delivery. Some authors have suggested that if delivery is planned before 38 weeks then fetal lung maturity should first be assessed by measurement of the lecithin–sphingomyelin ratio or phosphatidyl glycerol concentration in amniotic fluid obtained by amniocentesis. If there is a pressing clinical need to deliver prematurely, then the indication or indications alone should justify the intervention. On the other hand, if there is no overwhelming reason to terminate the pregnancy then no action should be taken. Amniocentesis was abandoned in Oxford in 1980 and we have since this time aimed to deliver all uncomplicated diabetic pregnancies at a minimum of 273 days (39 completed weeks) gestation.

In recent years some have advocated even later delivery at 40 weeks or after (Murphy et al 1984). These authors claimed that with an increase in mean gestational age from 37.4 to 39.4 weeks perinatal mortality was not altered, morbidity was reduced, and spontaneous vaginal deliveries increased from 14.3% to 37.8%. There was, however, a significant increase in birthweight from 3090 to 3650 g and one 39-week stillbirth in the 44 women delivered at term compared with none in the 35 women with earlier delivery.

Management of labour

Spontaneous vaginal delivery is one of the main aims in the modern management of the pregnant diabetic woman. An elective Caesarean section may, however, be indicated with fetal malpresentations, an estimated fetal weight in excess of 4.5 kg or a history of a previous Caesarean section. The use of intravenous therapy during labour inevitably limits the mobility of the diabetic woman but this inconvenience can be minimized by using battery-powered infusion equipment. Continuous fetal heart rate and contraction monitoring is advised because of the increased incidence of fetal distress in labour (Olofsson et al 1986), which may be due to an impaired maternal oxygen release in the utero-placental circulation (Madsen & Ditzel 1984). This can also be achieved, without appreciable loss of mobility, using modern telemetry equipment.

Provision of pain relief in labour is particularly important because painful uterine contractions cause catecholamine release, which in turn causes glycogenolysis and hyperglycaemia. Epidural anaesthesia is ideal but not vital, especially in the multiparous patient who may have a rapid and uncomplicated labour. If intravenous fluids are required for 'preloading' prior to insertion of an epidural or for the administration of oxytocin, it is essential that normal saline or Hartmann's solution and not dextrose is used in order to avoid fetal hyperglycaemia, as this predisposes to neonatal hypoglycaemia (see above).

The labour should always be supervised by senior midwifery and medical staff — preferably those with prior experience of the management of diabetes. This will be reassuring to the mother and avoid needless anxiety, which may have an adverse effect on the course of labour. Events during labour should be carefully recorded on a partogram and special attention must be given to the intravenous fluid load administered. Detailed records of the progress of labour are obligatory and the possible need for delivery by Caesarean section must be considered early in the labour if progress is poor or the fetus appears to be macrosomic on clinical or ultrasound assessment. Efforts to predict fetal macrosomia and in particular the risk of shoulder dystocia have, however, been conspicuously unsuccessful to date. Attempts to measure the biacromial diameter of the shoulders using computed tomography (Kitzmiller et al 1987) and magnetic resonance imaging appear promising for this purpose but are as yet rather unrefined. Using a shoulder width of 14 cm as a cut-off and a birthweight of 4.2 kg as an abnormal result Kitzmiller and co-workers (1987), however, showed that the predictive value of a positive test was 78% and of a negative test 100%.

The puerperium and contraception

Diabetics are at increased risk of wound infection following surgery, and prophylactic antibiotics are therefore advised following both elective and emergency Caesarean section.

Breast-feeding is encouraged. This reduces the insulin requirement by approximately 25% (Alban Davies et al 1989) and an appropriate reduction in dose should therefore be made in all these women once lactation is established. Women who choose not to breast-feed or in whom breast-feeding is unsuccessful should resume their prepregnancy insulin dose after delivery.

All diabetic women should be seen for a 6-week postnatal examination and offered contraceptive advice at this time. This will of course depend on the age, parity and future reproductive plans of each woman. The progestogen only (mini) pill has virtually no effect on carbohydrate or lipid metabolism. It is therefore suitable for the breast-feeding diabetic woman, and provided she is prepared to accept the slightly higher failure rate associated with this method when ovulation resumes, it may be used long term. The potentially adverse effects on carbohydrate and lipoprotein metabolism of the older high-dose combined oral contraceptive pills have long been a source of concern in diabetics. Recent data, however, suggest that modern low-dose preparations containing 'third-generation' progestogens have little effect on high or low-density lipoprotein concentrations or carbohydrate metabolism and can be used safely, especially in younger insulin-dependent and gestational diabetics. Early concerns about the apparently high failure rates of copper-containing intrauterine devices in diabetics have also been refuted in recent studies (Skouby et al 1991). Finally, the woman who has completed her family should be encouraged to consider a laparoscopic sterilization.

The Oxford experience: 1980–1990

During the 11-year period from 1 January 1980 to 31 December 1990 there were 270 insulin-treated pregnancies in 227 Oxford women, of whom 172 were insulin-dependent diabetics prior to the pregnancy. The remaining 98 pregnancies occurred in women who were diagnosed as gestational diabetics during the pregnancy and were treated with insulin because of persistent preprandial blood glucose concentrations in excess of 6.0 mmol/l despite dietary advice. The patient characteristics are shown in Table 3.5. A large number of the pregnancies in both groups went to term and some uncomplicated pregnancies were allowed to progress beyond 40 weeks, especially when the woman was particularly anxious to have a spontaneous onset labour.

During the 11-year period there were 2 stillbirths and 1 neonatal death — a perinatal mortality of 11.1 per 1000 total births. Two of these were potentially avoidable. The first in 1982 was of a grossly small-for-dates baby (<3rd centile) at 34 weeks, and the second at 38 weeks in a severely depressed patient who, despite advice, ignored reduced and subsequently absent fetal movements for 7 days. The single neonatal death occurred within 24 hours of delivery in 1985 and was due to transposition of the great vessels. This patient had neglected her diabetes both before conceiving and during the first trimester. She subsequently became obsessional about her control and delivered a healthy infant in 1987. Two pregnancies were terminated at 20 and 26 weeks, respectively, the former because of renal agenesis, the latter because of multiple congenital anomalies. Both were diagnosed during ultrasound anomaly scans.

The indications for induction of labour are shown in Table 3.6. The majority were performed because the patients had reached a gestation of 273 days. Spontaneous labour occurred in 33.7% of the insulin-dependent diabetics and 47.8% of the insulin-treated gestational diabetics.

Although our goal was to achieve vaginal deliveries whenever possible, nearly 50% of the insulin-dependent diabetics and just over a third of the insulin-treated gestational diabetics were delivered by Caesarean section (Table 3.7). This was in part due to the large number of women who had previously been delivered by Caesarean section, especially in the insulin-dependent diabetic group, but also reflects the phenomenon of 'obstetrician's distress' which occurs in diabetic labours where there is poor progress and the obstetrician becomes understandably anxious about the possibility of impending shoulder dystocia! It should be noted, in this context, that nearly a third (30.9%) of all the Caesarean sections in the insulin-dependent diabetic group were performed for cephalopelvic disproportion or the less firm diagnosis of

Table 3.5 Characteristics of the Oxford patients (1980–1991)

	Insulin-dependent ($n = 172$)		Insulin-treated gestational ($n = 98$)	
Age (years)	27.4	(5.1)	29.1	(5.6)
Weight at booking (kg)	65.3	(9.5)	71.0	(17.4)
Weight gain/week (kg)	0.51	(0.33)	0.39	(0.23)
Height (cm)	162.4	(6.8)	160.3	(6.3)
Gestation at delivery (weeks)	38.2	(1.9)	38.3	(2.1)
Birthweight (g)	3250	(657)	3378	(613)
Inpatient days	19.2	(0–213)	21.4	(4–88)

Table 3.6   Indications for induction of labaour

	Insulin-dependent (n = 93)	Insulin-treated gestational (n = 52)
Diabetes	69 (74.2%)	43 (82.7%)
Pre-eclampsia	10 (10.8%)	3 (5.8%)
Previous Caesarean section	5 (5.4%)	1 (1.9%)
Ruptured membranes	4 (4.3%)	2 (3.9%)
Intrauterine growth retardation	2 (2.1%)	1 (1.9%)
Intrauterine death	2 (2.1%)	—
Macrosomia	1 (1.1%)	—
Hypertension	—	1 (1.9%)
Social	—	1 (1.9%)

Table 3.7   Mode of delivery

	Insulin-dependent (n = 172)	Insulin-treated gestational (n = 98)
Spontaneous	58 (33.7%)	47 (48.0%)
Breech	2 (1.2%)	—
Forceps	29 (16.8%)	16 (16.3%)
Ventouse	2 (1.2%)	1 (1.0%)
Caesarean section	81 (47.1%)	34 (34.7%)

'poor progress' in labour, while no less than 42% of the insulin-treated gestational diabetics were delivered for these combined indications (Table 3.8).

Table 3.8   Indications for Caesarean section

	Insulin-dependent (n = 81)	Insulin-treated gestational (n = 34)
Previous Caesarean section	24 (29.7%)	11 (32.4%)
Poor progress in labour	19 (23.5%)	10 (29.4%)
Fetal distress in labour	17 (21.0%)	4 (11.8%)
Cephalopelvic disproportion	6 (7.4%)	4 (11.8%)
Breech	4 (4.9%)	1 (2.9%)
Pre-eclampsia	7 (8.6%)	—
Ruptured membranes	2 (2.5%)	—
Intrauterine growth retardation	—	2 (5.9%)
Placenta praevia	1 (1.2%)	—
Cord prolapse	—	1 (2.9%)
Failed forceps	1 (1.2%)	1 (2.9%)

We do *not* routinely admit the newborn infant to the special care nursery as this is usually not necessary. The infant remains with its mother and is fed early. Hourly blood glucose measurements are performed during the first 4 hours after delivery and careful observations are made to ensure there is no evidence of transient tachypnoea or the respiratory distress syndrome. In practice 48 (27.9%) of the infants of the insulin-dependent patients and 17 (17.3%) of the infants of the insulin-treated gestational diabetics were admitted to the special care nursery for observation or treatment.

KEY POINTS FOR CLINICAL PRACTICE

In conclusion, our scheme for 'success through simplicity' in diabetic pregnancy can be summarized as a 20-point plan, with ten 'medical' and ten 'obstetric' practice points.

Medical practice points

1. Ensure prepregnancy counselling
2. Arrange early antenatal booking
3. Advise blood glucose series at least twice weekly using a meter
4. Use human insulin
5. Frequent antenatal attendances (every 2 weeks until 32 weeks, then weekly)
6. Provide glucagon
7. Check the retinae
8. Aim for outpatient care
9. Use intravenous insulin and glucose infusions in labour
10. Reduce insulin to the prepregnancy dose after delivery.

Obstetric practice points

1. Early ultrasound dating scan
2. Anomaly ultrasound at 19 weeks
3. Fetal growth (head and abdominal circumference scans) at alternate visits
4. Weekly or twice-weekly biophysical profile scans from 36 weeks until delivery
5. Deliver at 273 days (39 completed weeks)
6. Aim for a vaginal delivery
7. Continuous fetal heart monitoring in labour
8. Ensure adequate analgesia in labour
9. Do not admit the baby routinely to the special care nursery
10. Encourage breast-feeding.

ACKNOWLEDGEMENT

The authors acknowledge with thanks the contributions made by Beryl M. Barringer SRD, Dietitian, and K. Vibeke Mannion SRN, RSCN, SCM and Tansy M. Cheston RGN, RM, Specialist Midwives, John Radcliffe Maternity

Hospital, Oxford, to the development of policy and views expressed in this chapter.

REFERENCES

Alban Davies H, Clark J D A, Dalton K J, Edwards O M 1989 Insulin requirements of women who breast feed. Br Med J 298: 1357–1358

Ales K L, Santini D L 1989 Should all pregnant women be screened for gestational glucose intolerance? Lancet i: 1187–1191

Barnett A H, Stubbs S M, Mander A M 1980 Management of premature labour in diabetic pregnancy. Diabetologia 18: 365–368

Barss V A 1989 Obstetrical complications. In Hare J W (ed) Diabetes complicating pregnancy. Liss, New York, pp 125–134

Cousins L 1987 Pregnancy complications among diabetic women. Review 1965–1985. Obstet Gynecol Surv 42: 140–149

Coustan D R 1991 Maternal insulin to lower the risk of fetal macrosomia in diabetic pregnancy. Clin Obstet Gynecol 34: 288–295

Delaney J J, Ptacek J 1970 Three decades of experience with diabetic pregnancies. Am J Obstet Gynecol 106: 550–556

Duncan J M 1883 On puerperal diabetes. Trans Obstet Soc London 24: 256–285

Gregory R, Tattersall R B 1992 Are diabetic pre-pregnancy clinics worthwhile? Lancet 340: 656–657

Fog-Pedersen J, Molsted-Pedersen L 1989 Ultrasound studies on fetal growth. In: Sutherland H W, Stowers J M, Pearson D W M (eds) Carbohydrate metabolism in pregnancy and the newborn IV. Springer-Verlag, Berlin, pp 83–93

Gabbe S G 1980 Medical complications of pregnancy. Management of diabetes in pregnancy: six decades of experience. In: Pitkin R M, Zlatnik F J (eds) Year book of obstetrics and gynecology. Year Book Medical Publishers, Chicago, pp 37–49

Garner P R, D'Alton M E, Dudley D K et al 1990 Preeclampsia in diabetic pregnancies. Am J Obstet Gynecol 163: 505–508

Gillmer, M D G, Beard R W 1975 Fetal and placental function tests in diabetic pregnancy. In: Sutherland H W, Stowers J M (eds) Carbohydrate metabolism in pregnancy and the newborn. Churchill Livingstone, Edinburgh, 168–194

Green J R, Pawson I G, Schumacher L B et al 1990 Glucose tolerance in pregnancy: Ethnic variation and influence of body habitus. Am J Obstet Gynecol 163: 86–92

Greene M F, Hare J W, Krache M et al 1989 Prematurity among insulin requiring diabetic gravid women. Am J Obstet Gynecol 161: 106–111

Hadden D R 1989 The first recorded case of diabetic pregnancy (Bennewitz H G, 1824, University of Berlin). Diabetologia 32: 625

Hare J W 1991 Complicated diabetes complicating pregnancy. Clin Obstet Gynecol 5: 349–367

Johnson J M, Lange I R, Harman C R et al 1988 Biophysical profile scoring in the management of the diabetic pregnancy. Obstet Gynecol 72: 841–846

Johnstone F D, Steel J M, Haddad N G et al 1992 Doppler umbilical artery flow velocity waveforms in diabetic pregnancy. Br J Obstet Gynaecol 99: 135–140

Jovanovic L, Peterson C M 1983 Insulin requirements during the first stage of labor in insulin-dependent diabetic women. Am J Med 75: 607–612

Karlsson K, Kjellmer L 1972 The outcome of diabetic pregnancies in relation to the mother's blood sugar level. Am J Obstet Gynecol 112: 213–220

Kitzmiller J L, Mall J C, Gin G D et al 1987 Measurement of shoulder width with computed tomography in diabetic women. Obstet Gynecol 70: 941–945

Landon M B, Gabbe S G, Bruner J P, Ludmir J 1989 Doppler umbilical artery velocimetry in pregnancy complicated by insulin-dependent diabetes mellitus. Am J Obstet Gynecol 163: 1040–1048

Langer O, Levy J, Brustman L et al 1989 Glycaemic control in gestational diabetes mellitus. How tight is tight enough: small for gestational age versus large for gestational age? Am J Obstet Gynecol 161: 646–653

Lind T 1985 Antenatal screening using random blood glucose values. Diabetes 34 Suppl

2: 17–20

Lind T, Phillips P R 1991 Influence of pregnancy on the 75 g OGTT: a prospective multicenter study. Diabetes 40/Suppl 2: 8–13

Lufkin E G, Nelson R L, Hill L M 1984 An analysis of pregnancies at Mayo Clinic, 1950–79. Diabetes Care 7: 539–547

Madsen H, Ditzel J 1984 Red cell 2,3-diphosphoglycerate and haemoglobin-oxygen affinity during diabetic pregnancy. Acta Obstet Gynecol Scand 63: 403–406

McFarland K F, Case C A 1985 The relationship of maternal age on gestational diabetes. Diabetes Care 8: 598–600

Manning F A, Baskett T F, Morrison I, Lange I 1981 Fetal biophysical profile scoring: a prospective study in 1,184 high risk patients. Am J Obstet Gynecol 140: 289–294

Manning F A 1990 The fetal biophysical score: current status. Obstet Gynecol Clin North Am 17: 147–162

Maran A, Lomas J, Archibald H et al 1993 Double blind clinical and laboratory study of hypoglycaemia with human and porcine insulin in diabetic patients reporting hypoglycaemia unawareness after transferring to human insulin. Br Med J 306: 167–171

Menon R K, Cohen R M, Sperling M A et al 1990 Transplacental passage of insulin in pregnant women with insulin-dependent diabetes mellitus: its role in fetal macrosomia. N Eng J Med 323: 309–315

Miodovnik M, Peros N, Holroyde J C, Siddiqi T A 1985 Treatment of premature labor in insulin-dependent diabetic women. Obstet Gynecol 65: 621–627

Mohen D, Newnham J P, D'Orsogna L 1992 Indomethacin for the treatment of polyhydramnios: a case of constriction of the ductus arteriosus. Aust NZ J Obstet Gynecol 32: 243–246

Moise K J 1991 Indomethacin therapy in the treatment of symptomatic polyhydramnios. Clin Obstet Gynecol 34: 310–318

Murphy J, Peters J, Morris P et al 1984 Conservative management of pregnancy in diabetic women. Br Med J 288: 1203–1205

Olofsson P, Ingemarsson I, Solum T 1986 Fetal distress during labour in diabetic pregnancy. Br J Obstet Gynecol 93: 1067–1071

O'Sullivan J B, Mahan C M 1964 Criteria for the oral glucose tolerance test in pregnancy. Diabetes 13: 278–285

O'Sullivan J B, Mahan C M, Charles D, Dandrow R V 1973 Screening criteria for high risk gestational diabetic patients. Am J Obstet Gynecol 116: 895–900

O'Sullivan J B 1991 Diabetes mellitus after GDM. Diabetes 40 Suppl 2: 131–135

Pettitt D J, Knowler W C, Baird H R, Bennett P H 1990 Gestational diabetes: infant and maternal complications of pregnancy in relation to third trimester glucose tolerance in the Pima Indians. Diabetes Care 3: 458–464

Proceedings of the Second International Workshop Conference on Gestational Diabetes Mellitus 1985 Summary and Recommendations of the Second International Workshop Conference on Gestational Diabetes Mellitus. Diabetes 34 Suppl 2: 123–126

Roberts M F, Neff K, Hubbell J P et al 1976 Association between maternal disease and the respiratory distress syndrome in the new born. N Eng J Med 294: 357–360

Roberts A B, Baker J R, Metcalf P, Mullard C 1990 Fructosamine compared with a glucose load as a screening test for gestational diabetes. Obstet Gynecol 76: 773–775

Shir M M 1939 Diabetes in pregnancy with observations in 28 cases. Am J Obstet Gynecol 37: 1032–1035

Skipper E 1933 Diabetes mellitus and pregnancy: a clinical and analytical study. Q J Med 2: 353–80

Skouby S O, Molsted-Pedersen L, Petersen K R 1991 Contraception for women with diabetes: an update. Clin Obstet Gynecol 5: 493–503

Soler N G, Walsh C H, Malins J M 1978 Neonatal morbidity among infants of diabetic mothers. Q J Med 45: 303–313

Spellacy W N 1969 Diabetes complicating pregnancy. Mod Med 37: 91–102

Titus R S 1937 Diabetes in pregnancy from the obstetric point of view. Am J Obstet Gynecol 33: 386–392

Wald N J, Cuckle H S, Densem J W, Stone R B 1992 Maternal serum unconjugated oestriol and human chorionic gonadotrophin levels in pregnancies with insulin-dependent diabetes: implications for screening for Down's syndrome. Br J Obstet Gynecol 99: 51–53

Williams J W 1909 The clinical significance of glycosuria in pregnant women. Am J Med Sci
137: 1–26
WHO Expert Committee on Diabetes Mellitus (1980) World Health Organization Technical
Report Series 646
Yudkin J S, Knopfler A 1992 Glucose and insulin infusions during labour. Br Med J
339: 1479

Appendix: Printouts from Ames memory meter and 'intelligent' printer

GLUCOMETER®M DATA SUMMARY

Copyright (c) 1986 Miles Laboratories, Inc.
GLUCOFACTS Data Printer   Version 1.00

Name :   ID :

Data from 28 May to 10 Jun   LAST 14 DAYS SELECTED

Current Date :   Physician :

STATISTICS

Number of Days Covered 14
Number of Readings Done 91
Average Number Readings/Day 6.5

Average Blood Glucose .... 5.0 mmol/L

20% of Readings at or Below .... 3.1 mmol/L
20% of Readings at or Above .... 7.2 mmol/L

Lowest Blood Glucose .... 1.4 mmol/L
Highest Blood Glucose .... 13.3 mmol/L

Printout 1 Patient details and statistics.

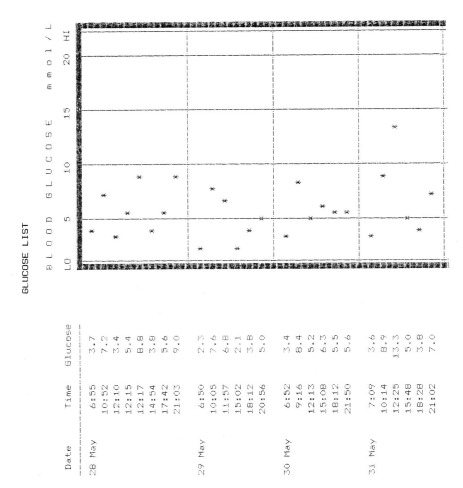

Printout 2   Individual starved times and blood glucose measurements.

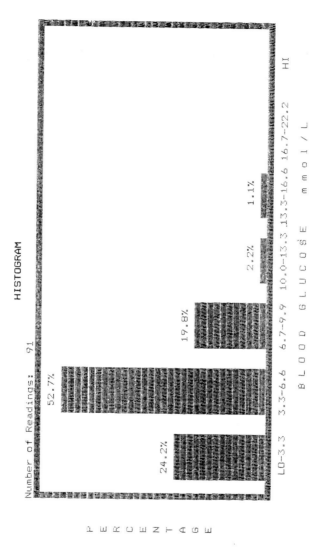

Printout 3   Histogram of blood glucose values.

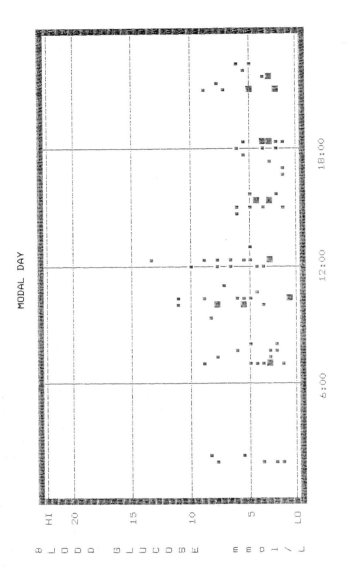

Printout 4   Summation of blood glucose values in a 'modal day'.

4

Advances in the diagnosis and management of fetal distress in labour

G. J. Mires   N. B. Patel

What is fetal distress?

The term 'fetal distress' is widely used in obstetric practice, but is a term which lacks a precise definition. It has variously been applied to labours complicated by fetal heart rate pattern abnormalities or meconium staining of the liquor, the presence of mild umbilical arterial acidaemia or infants with low Apgar scores. In all of these cases a poor association with subsequent adverse neurological outcome has been demonstrated, and there has been growing concern about electronic fetal monitoring as Caesarean section rates have risen with a failure to demonstrate any clear benefits in terms of perinatal mortality and long-term outcome (Sykes et al 1982, Low et al 1983, Dijxhoorn et al 1985, Ruth & Raivio 1988, MacDonald et al 1985). This makes the evaluation of intrapartum fetal monitoring by appropriate end points confusing and often misleading. In obstetric terms, however, the aim of intrapartum fetal monitoring remains the identification of events which if continued would result in fetal damage or death; the methods employed to identify these events should have sufficient sensitivity and positive predictive values to allow intervention before the onset of permanent fetal damage. In pathophysiological terms, cellular damage due to hypoxia occurs as a consequence of comprise to cellular central metabolism. A normal fetus is well adapted to the intermittent hypoxia occurring during normal labour by switching to periods of anaerobic metabolism and redistributing blood to vital organs such as the brain and myocardium. However, during periods of prolonged oxygen reduction the fetal buffering system cannot maintain a normal pH as increased organic acids such as lactic acid are produced by anaerobic metabolism, and this results in the development of a metabolic acidosis. In view of these pathophysiological changes occurring in response to hypoxia and resulting in cell damage, current techniques for intrapartum assessment are therefore targeted towards the direct or indirect measurement of fetal acid/base status or fetal oxygenation.

This chapter will review the available techniques, recent advances in the development of new monitoring techniques and ways in which obstetric management will be influenced by their use.

The current intrapartum monitoring techniques

Fetal heart rate monitoring, scalp pH and meconium staining of amniotic fluid

In 1963 Caldeyro-Barcia et al performed the original work detailing fetal heart range changes in response to uterine contractions. Monitoring anencephalic fetuses, they observed that if late decelerations had occurred for some time, fetal death occurred. Subsequently, electronic monitoring was rapidly introduced and has been the standard technique used to 'diagnose' fetal distress for the past two decades. The findings of a survey in the USA in 1980 revealed that 48% of births had continuous electronic fetal heart rate monitoring performed. Since its widespread introduction, several studies have demonstrated that abnormal fetal heart rate tracings do not correlate well with poor fetal outcome and have failed to confirm the benefits suggested by early retrospective analyses. Electronic fetal monitoring therefore shows great sensitivity but poor specificity and positive predictive value in correlating fetal distress as defined by an abnormal fetal heart rate pattern with subsequent adverse neonatal outcome, but does, however, continue to give obstetricians much comfort in the fact that a completely normal trace prior to delivery is associated with good fetal outcome in 99% of cases (Zuspan et al 1979, Haverkamp et al 1976, Kelso et al 1978, Thacker 1987, Boehm 1990). The reading, classification and interpretation of fetal heart rate recordings is subject to considerable inter-observer and even intra-observer variation, and the fetal outcome depends both on the correct interpretation of the data and appropriate action by the attending staff. Dawes et al (1992) and Cheung et al (1992) have published their results for the use of computerized antenatal cardiotocographic (CTG) assessment. They conclude that computerized assessment agrees closely with experienced visual assessment, especially where that assessment depends on the estimation of fetal heart rate variation when visual analysis was found to be unreliable. The extension of this work to the intrapartum period may improve the specificity of the CTG in labour.

The monitoring of fetal heart rate during labour remains the mainstay of intrapartum fetal assessment, either continually with electronic fetal monitoring or by intermittent auscultation, but because of its poor specificity for identifying fetal compromise an increased incidence of instrumental deliveries has been noted, with no measurable improvement in fetal outcome (Haverkamp et al 1979).

Fetal blood sampling was introduced to recognize those infants developing acidosis when a non-reassuring fetal heart rate pattern is encountered, in an attempt to reduce unnecessary obstetric intervention in monitored pregnancies. Scalp sampling is, however, only practised in 50% of consultant units in the UK (Wheble et al 1989). It has become accepted that a fetal scalp pH of <7.20 indicates fetal compromise, but although 30% of these infants are depressed at birth, most are vigorous and show no short or long-term sequelae (Tucker & Hauth 1990). Severe acidaemia does correlate with an increased incidence of neonatal seizures and hypotonia, and the identification of a developing acidosis especially with a metabolic component and subsequent appropriate obstetric intervention is likely to reduce the incidence of these complications. The validity of scalp capillary measurements as the head is compresssed against the pelvis has, however, been questioned (O'Connor et al 1979).

The third conventional parameter for the identification of fetal compromise is the presence of meconium-stained amniotic fluid. Approximately 20% of babies will pass meconium during labour, particularly post-dates pregnancies, but heavy meconium has been associated with severe or repeated stress (Meis et al 1978).

In association with an abnormal fetal heart rate pattern, the presence of meconium is often used as an indication for fetal blood sampling (Miller et al 1975). The presence of meconium-stained liquor has not, however, been demonstrated to correlate with adverse neurological sequelae (Nelson & Ellenberg 1984, Dijxhoorn et al 1986).

The poor specificity and predictive value of the available intrapartum monitoring techniques have led to the need for more reliable methods of fetal monitoring in labour (Sawers 1983). These new approaches include the fetal electrocardiogram (FECG), continuous tissue pH, transcutaneous pCO_2 and pO_2, near-infrared spectroscopy and pulse oximetry.

FETAL ELECTROCARDIOGRAM

The derivation of the fetal heart rate from the R–R interval of the FECG is only one segment of the information available from the ECG waveform. Initial subjective assessment of the ECG changes was considered to be too crude to be of value in the intrapartum assessment of fetal compromise, and problems associated with signal noise made the FECG unpopular as a monitoring technique. However, with the advent of computer systems and the associated improved technology, interest has been shown in its use during the intrapartum period.

Hypoxia and acidaemia induced in exteriorized fetal lambs and guinea pigs by Rosen & Kjellmer (1975) produced changes in the ST segment and T wave, with a progressive increase in the T wave amplitude. These changes occurred before signs of cardiovascular failure (Rosen et al 1976). The changes observed in the ST segment were correlated to the anaerobic breakdown of myocardial glycogen stores (Rosen & Isaksson 1976) and could be reproduced by β-adrenoceptor stimulation (Hokegard et al 1979). Elevation of the T/QRS ratio is therefore considered to represent a change in anaerobic myocardial metabolism (Greene et al 1982) and offers a means by which myocardial adaptation to hypoxia might be identified (Rosen 1986).

Lilja et al (1985) reported the results of ST waveform changes on the FECG in a clinical study of 46 patients. The FECG was obtained with a conventional fetal scalp electrode. Although no infant was clinically hypoxic

(5 min Apgar <7) only 26% of the patients studied had a continuously normal CTG, whereas 67% had no ST waveform abnormalities. A linear relationship was found between T/QRS ratio before birth and cord plasma lactate values, but no correlation was identified between T/QRS ratio and umbilical cord arterial pH. Greene et al (1982) demonstrated, however, that raised lactate levels precede a fall in pH by some hours during hypoxia in chronic fetal lambs, secondary to the buffering mechanisms, and hence changes in T/QRS ratio may represent an earlier means of identifying hypoxia.

Jenkins et al (1986) reported the results of ST segment change in 24 fetuses, 14 of whom were non-acidotic and 10 of whom were acidotic at delivery. They found a highly significant correlation between both a long-term increase in ST segment and T wave height and fetal acidosis. In their group, 9 of the 10 acidotic infants had ST segment and T wave changes giving a sensitivity of 90%, specificity 87% and a positive predictive value of 82% for ST segment changes predicting acidosis at delivery. They commented that these figures were based on a small number of cases, and that the potential for overcoming the currrent difficulties in intrapartum fetal monitoring using this technique was promising.

Johanson et al (1992) found that in labours in whom continuous electronic fetal heart rate monitoring was being performed, and in whom a non-reassuring trace was obtained, the fetal ECG by assessment of the T/QRS ratio provided independent information from heart rate, and that this information could be useful in separating physiological from pathological CTG traces. They felt that this might reduce the need for fetal blood sampling.

Similarly in a study by Arulkumaran et al (1990) the specificity of the T/QRS ratio to identify fetuses at risk of metabolic acidosis was reported to be increased when combined with fetal heart rate changes. The Plymouth Perinatal Research Group have produced clinical guidelines for action in the mature fetus based on CTG analysis and ST waveform changes for use with the commercially available ST analyser (STAN) and used in their randomized trial (see later). This group emphasize, however, that changes in ST patterns should always be interpreted in conjunction with the CTG patterns.

Maclachlan et al (1992) recently reported on a study of fetal acidaemia, the T/QRS ratio and the CTG, and found that a raised T/QRS ratio had a considerably lower detection rate than the pathological CTG for fetal acidaemia during labour. Murphy et al (1992) reported no correlation between T/QRS ratio and umbilical artery pH or Apgar scores. Newbold et al (1991) also reported similar negative findings regarding the relationship between the T/QRS ratio and metabolic acidosis. The numbers in these studies were small, however, and all groups emphasize the need for larger trials such as the multicentre European Community trial currently in progress, as reiterated by Lilja et al (1989). This group used a microprocessor to analyse the FECG and produced data which indicated that dynamic ST waveform changes also occur during the delivery of non-asphyxiated children;

they concluded that no absolute statement should be made on the role of ST waveform analysis in fetal monitoring as long as the material does not include data from asphyxiated children.

As one of the major shortcomings of intrapartum CTG monitoring is poor specificity for detecting birth asphyxia, a potential role of the intrapartum FECG might be to improve this specificity — a role supported by the experimental and clinical data. Used in conjunction with the CTG, Westgate et al (1992) were the first to publish the results from a randomized prospective controlled trial studying intervention rates and neonatal outcome for high-risk labours monitored either by conventional CTG or by ST waveform analysis in addition to CTG monitoring using the STAN monitor. The addition of ECG waveform analysis was associated with significantly fewer operative deliveries for fetal distress with no significant difference in neonatal outcome. The lower intervention rates occurred among those cases where the CTG pattern was classified as normal or intermediate. There was no significant difference in the intervention rates among cases with abnormal CTG recordings. A further observation from this study was that a negative T wave and/or ST depression should be regarded as abnormal even although the T/QRS ratio may not be raised and may be negative.

As well as changes in the T/QRS ratio, Murray (1986) observed that the usually positive correlation between P–R interval and the R–R interval is reversed in the presence of falling scalp or umbilical pH, and a shortened P–R interval is observed despite slowing of the heart rate. This may be a means of differentiating fetal heart rate decelerations produced by reflex non-hypoxic increases in vagal tone from those secondary to hypoxia, metabolically mediated through the sympathetic system.

If the ECG waveform is to be of use as an indicator of fetal well-being, then a multivariant analysis such as ST changes in association with correlation of the P–R interval and R–R interval may well be necessary. However, it is important that proper assessment of this new technique is made in large trials which include asphyxiated infants prior to its introduction into routine clinical practice. The full significance of some of the ECG changes occurring during labour remains unclear.

INTRAPARTUM CONTINUOUS FETAL TISSUE PH MEASUREMENTS

Using a combined glass reference electrode, Stamm et al (1974) was the first to perform tissue pH measurements in the newborn, and a modification of this electrode was used for clinical trials involving the human fetus. The value of continuous fetal tissue pH measurements over intermittent fetal blood sampling is that a continuous assessment of pH allows the obstetrician to use acid/base information to asssess fetal metabolism during labour, provides an early warning of hypoxia, and avoids repeated amnioscopy. Close correlation has been found between tissue pH and capillary blood pH measured from the scalp (Stamm et al 1974). Chatterjee & Hochberg (1991) found that a poor neonatal outcome was predicted more reliably when the tissue pH was acidotic than by the acidotic capillary pH.

The glass electrodes currently available have a high rate of unsuccessful recordings, require sterilization and time-consuming calibration, are subject to breakage and have a limited life. This makes the technique expensive. More recently, however, a fibreoptic pH electrode has become available but Hochberg et al (1988) reported a success rate of only 80% with its use.

The disadvantages of the technique are therefore that the procedure is invasive and expensive. Although newer pH electrodes appear encouraging with respect to practicality and reliability, their usefulness remains unproven.

CONTINUOUS FETAL TRANSCUTANEOUS OXYGEN AND CARBON DIOXIDE TENSION

Transcutaneous oxygen tension ($tcpO_2$) and carbon dioxide tension ($tcpCO_2$) can both be measured using a superficially applied pO_2/pCO_2 electrode attached to the fetal scalp with a specifically designed suction ring. As with the tissue pH measurements, however, this technique is associated with numerous factors which may adversely influence the recordings. The so-called 'tonsure' effect (O'Connor et al 1979), the development of caput succedaneum (Lofgren & Jacobson 1977) or pressure of the electrode on the bony pelvis can result in inaccurate recording of both $tcpO_2$ and $tcpCO_2$.

Smits et al (1989), by measuring scalp blood flow using Doppler ultrasound and simultaneous $tcpO_2$ during labour, found that the $tcpO_2$ value was considerably influenced by local scalp blood flow and was therefore a questionable parameter. As with the tissue pH electrode, successful recordings can be anticipated in approximately 80% of cases (Weber 1979, Okane et al 1989). In association with this, only weak associations have been reported between $tcpO_2$ and umbilical arterial pO_2 levels (O'Connor & Hytten 1979, Weber 1979).

This technique has, however, been reported to aid in the management of cases of fetal arrhythmia, e.g. premature beats or paroxysmal supraventricular tachycardia when fetal heart rate monitoring during labour is not possible (van der Berg et al 1989, 1991)

PULSE OXIMETRY

Pulse oximetry is a non-invasive technique which has been extensively used by anaesthetists and neonatologists to monitor continuously arterial oxygen saturation. Because adult and neonatal sensors rely on the transmission of light through tissues, until recent modifications (Johnson et al 1991) fetal applications have not been possible.

Oximetry utilizes the fact that the light absorption spectra of oxygenated and reduced haemoglobins differ. Two reference wavelengths are used — one in the red and one in the near-infrared — and by considering the ratio of the two pulsatile (vascular bed) components (red/infrared) the percentage of saturated haemoglobin can be calculated. By calculating the ratio at the peaks of the pulsatile signal, the pulse oximeter indicates the oxygen saturation levels of arterial blood (SaO_2). In the oximeter sensor, red and infrared light-emitting diodes are in a bed of carbon paint to prevent light shunting across the probe, and the probe is placed above the cervix on the presenting part of the fetus at a low suction pressure, which ensures apposition.

Oxygenation and acidosis are related to fetal well-being, and specific advantages of recording SaO_2 rather than partial pressure of oxygen (PaO_2) have been reported. These include: (a) for the oxygen pressure electrode the need for frequent calibration and the problem of shift associated with the requirement of firm fixation techniques and local heating, which can result in scalp burns, with these problems not being associated with the pulse oximeter; (b) the observation that small changes in PaO_2 result in large changes in SaO_2 according to the oxygen dissociation curve, with these large changes in SaO_2 being easier to measure accurately than the small changes in PaO_2; and (c) the Bohr effect, resulting in a shift of the oxygen dissociation curve to the right, with increased hydrogen ion concentration and increased 2,3-diphosphoglycerate levels and the possibility of an acidotic fetus having a normal PaO_2 but a low SaO_2.

Initial reports on the use of pulse oximeters during labour are encouraging. Johnson et al (1991) successfully monitored 86 labours and reported a fall in oxygen saturation as labour progressed, from 68% (SD 13%) in early labour to 58% (SD 17%) at the end of labour. More recently, McNamara et al (1992) reported a significant association between pulse oximetry readings, umbilical venous oxygen saturation and umbilical cord blood pH values.

Gardosi et al (1991) reported failure to obtain adequate readings in 44 of 105 labours, and indicated the recognition of the problems and limitations of this new application. Amongst them they suggest caput succedaneum due to false (non-arterial) pulse rate (Johnson et al 1990), inadequate probe contact, and substantial variation in the fetal/adult haemoglobin ratio amongst fetuses (Andrews & Willet 1965), which can affect the oxygen dissociation curve shift with reduction in pO_2. They conclude (Gardosi et al 1991) that pulse oximetry may become a potential adjunct to fetal heart rate monitoring. It can offer reassurance of fetal well-being non-invasively if a stable SaO_2 baseline is obtained, especially in the presence of a questionable fetal heart rate recording, and may reduce the need for fetal blood sampling. It may also assess fetal reserve with a low baseline SaO_2 at the start of labour, suggesting diminished placental transfer, and recognize fetal distress with a falling SaO_2 during labour, suggesting a developing metabolic acidosis.

NEAR-INFRARED SPECTROSCOPY

This is a new technique which is attracting a lot of interest, and may have the potential to allow cerebral hypoxia to be detected in the fetus during delivery. It is based on the principle that light will be absorbed by matter, and the amount absorbed will bear some relationship to the concentration of the substance responsible for the absorption. Jobis (1977) made the observation that using near-infrared it is possible to make measurements through relatively large tissue segments. The absorption spectra for oxygenated haemoglobin (HbO$_2$) and deoxygenated haemoglobin (Hb) are well established and it is theoretically possible to make measurements in deep tissue segments using near-infrared. The respiratory enzyme cytochrome aa$_3$, situated at the terminal end of the respiratory chain and responsible for donating electrons directly to oxygen molecules, has a broad absorption peak when oxidized in the near-infrared range (Rea et al 1985). Measurement of changes in intracellular oxygen utilization of large tissue masses is again therefore theoretically possible.

The use of this method in a clinical fetal application has significant theoretical and practical problems. Rolfe et al (1982) has demonstrated that probe attachment is not straightforward, although some success was achieved using suction or tissue adhesives. To obtain significant penetration of cerebral tissue, the fibres must be spaced by more than 4 cm, and to construct such fibres is difficult and the procedure becomes intrusive (Rolfe et al 1991). Recent probe designs do, however, appear more promising, and Schmidt et al (1991) using animal models have obtained signals providing information of the relative changes in haemoglobin concentration blood volume and cytochrome aa$_3$.

This technique therefore has great potential, but at present for fetal intrapartum monitoring it is limited by the lack of availability of the ideal fibre and probe design.

MANAGEMENT OF FETAL DISTRESS

Faced with the suspicion that fetal distress has developed during the first or second stage of labour, delivery of the fetus by Caesarean section is the adequate response in the first stage, and delivery by forceps, ventouse or in some cases Caesarean section in the second stage.

Fetal 'resuscitation' is an attractive proposition if the fetal condition is not deteriorating rapidly or if fetal distress is not severe. To date limited attention has been given to possible techniques to improve the condition of the fetus during labour. Current 'first-aid' manoeuvres include a change in maternal position and in particular avoidance of the supine position, stopping exogenous oxytocin administration, use of β-sympathomimetics and administration of oxygen. The use of saline amnio-infusion has also been addressed.

A change in maternal position may have a beneficial effect on the incidence and severity of fetal heart decelerations, especially if a fetal bradycardia is associated with an aortocaval occlusion. A dorsal position during the second stage of labour has been associated with a fall in umbilical arterial pH and elevated pCO_2 levels (Johnstone et al 1987).

Hyperstimulation of the uterus with exogenous oxytocin can result in fetal bradycardias, and Klink et al (1981) found a correlation between the $tcpCO_2$ and uterine contraction interval. A rapid response is noted on cessation of the oxytocin, and a single dose of ritodrine or terbutaline may relax the uterus sufficiently to reduce cord compression or increase uteroplacental blood flow (Shekerloo et al 1989).

The value of maternal inhalation of oxygen has been questioned, with a negative effect on intervillous blood flow being postulated (Jouppila et al 1983). Even using 100% oxygen despite significant increases in the maternal arterial pO_2 only a small increase in fetal arterial pO_2 is observed (Van Geijn et al 1991).

Saline amnio-infusion is a technique which has been advocated for relief of repetitive variable decelerations (Miyazaki & Nevarez & 1985) and the prevention of meconium aspiration (Wenstrom & Parsons 1989).

CONCLUSIONS

To the fetus labour is a stressful event, and in most instances it is well tolerated. The obstetrician faces the continual dilemma, however, of deciding in the face of currently available monitoring techniques which fetuses are stressed and which are distressed, with a hasty reaction leading to unnecessary obstetric intervention, and a tardy reaction or no reaction to the presence of fetal distress resulting in neonatal morbidity.

Current methods of assessment rely primarily on information gathered by CTG, and this lacks specificity. From the previous discussion it has been suggested that the use of fetal heart rate abnormalities, perhaps analysed by computer systems, and used in conjunction with other techniques such as FECG, pulse oximetry or continuous tissue pH monitoring, may improve the specificity and positive predictive value. These techniques will not be available or desirable for all labours, and methods of identifying labours at risk of developing fetal distress and in whom the use of these techniques would be applicable are required. Clinical risk factors have some predictive value but on their own lack precision, and there is no agreement amongst clinicians about the clinical factors which are of greatest use. Therefore, although clinical factors may contribute to a predictive score, it seems likely that the addition of biophysical methods will be required to achieve the precision needed for clinical practice. Both labour ward CTG and fetal breathing movements have been reported as being positively associated with metabolic acidaemia at delivery (Sasoon et al 1990), as has amniotic fluid volume. In our own studies in Dundee umbilical arterial Doppler within 7 days of delivery was also predictive of late decelerations in labour and admission of infants to the special care baby unit (SCBU) (Dempster et al 1988). Malcus et al (1991) found an association between abnormal umbilical arterial flow velocity waveforms in labour and umbilical arterial acidaemia, but not with CTG abnormalities. These factors may therefore form the basis of an intrapartum biophysical profile score to select which labours might benefit from the use of the newer and in some instances invasive and intrusive intrapartum monitoring techniques.

The intrapartum monitoring techniques discussed in this chapter all demonstrate promise in identifying various deviations in intrapartum acid/ base status and fetal oxygenation. Some of the techniques, such as tissue pH and near-infrared spectroscopy currently suffer from technical difficulties, but advances in technology are likely to overcome these problems. Other techniques such as FECG have overcome initial technical difficulties and now require evaluation in large clinical trials before introduction in routine obstetric practice.

No one technique is likely to provide the 'gold standard' in intrapartum assessment, and the maximum information on the fetus will be obtained by a combination of techniques. The appropriate selection of pregnancies on which to use the monitoring techniques remains a major challenge.

REFERENCES

Andrews B F, Willet G P 1965 Fetal haemoglobin concentration in the newborn. Am J Obstet Gynecol 91: 85–88
Arulkumaran S, Lilta H, Lindecrantz K et al 1990 Fetal ECG waveform analysis should improve fetal surveillance in labour. J Perinat Med 18: 13–22
Boehm F H 1990 Fetal distress. In: Eden R E, Boehm F H (eds) Assessment and care of the fetus: physiological, clinical and medicolegal principles. Prentice Hall, East Norwalk, pp 809–821
Caldeyro-Barcia R, Poseiro J, Negreiros de Pavia C et al 1963 Effects of abnormal uterine contractions on a human fetus. Bibl Paediatr 81: 267–295
Chatterjee M S, Hochberg H M 1991 Continuous intrapartum measurement of tissue pH of the human fetus using newly developed techniques. J Perinat Med 19: 93–96
Cheung L C, Gibb D M, Ajayi R A, Soothill P 1992 A comparison between computerised (mean range) and clinical visual cardiotocographic assessment. Br J Obstet Gynaecol 99: 817–820
Dawes G S, Lobb M, Moulden M et al 1992 Antenatal cardiotocogram quality and interpretation using computers. Br J Obstet Gynaecol 99: 791–797
Dempster J, Mires G J, Taylor D J et al 1988 Fetal umbilical artery flow velocity waveforms: prediction of SGA infants and late decelerations in labour. Eur J Obstet Gynecol Reprod Biol 29: 21–25
Dijxhoorn M J, Visser G H A, Huisjes P R et al 1985 The relationship between umbilical arteries pH, values and neonatal neurological morbidity in full term appropriate for dates infants. Early Hum Dev 11: 33–42
Dijxhoorn M J, Visser G, Fidler J J 1986 Apgar score, meconium and acidaemia at birth in relation to neonatal and neurological morbidity in term infants. Br J Obstet Gynaecol 93: 217–222
Gardosi J, Schram C M, Symonds E M 1991 Adaptation of pulse oximetry for fetal monitoring during labour. Lancet 327: 1265–1267
Greene K R, Dawes G S, Lilja H et al 1982 Changes in the ST waveform of the fetal ECG with hypoxemia. Am J Obstet Gynecol 144: 950–958
Haverkamp A D, Orleans M, Langendoerfer S et al 1979 A controlled trial of the differential effects of intrapartum fetal monitoring. Am J Obstet Gynecol 134: 399
Haverkamp A D, Thompson H E, McFee J G et al 1976 The evaluation of continuous fetal heart rate monitoring in high risk pregnanciess. Am J Obstet Gynecol 125: 310

Hochberg H M, Roby P V, Snell H M et al 1988 Continuous intrapartum fetal scalp pH and ECG monitoring by a fiberoptic probe. J Perinat Med 16 (Suppl 1): 71

Hokegard W H, Karlsson K, Kjellmer I et al 1979 ECG changes in the fetal lamb during asphyxia in relation to B adrenoceptor stimulation and blockade. Acta Physiol Scand 105: 195–203

Jenkins H M L, Symonds E M, Kirk D L et al 1986 Can fetal ECG improve the prediction of intrapartum fetal acidosis. Br J Obstet Gynaecol 93: 6–12

Jobis F F 1977 Non invasive infra red monitoring of cerebral and myocardial oxygen sufficiency and circulatory parameters. Science 98: 1264–1267

Johanson R B, Rice C, Shokr A et al 1992 ST-waveform analysis of the fetal ECG could reduce fetal blood sampling. Br J Obstet Gynaecol 99: 167–168

Johnson N, Johnson V, Banniseter J et al 1990 The effect of caput succedameum on oxygen saturation measurements. Br J Obstet Gynaecol 19: 493–498

Johnson N, Johnson V, Fisher S et al 1991 Fetal monitoring with pulse oximetry. Br J Obstet Gynaecol 98: 36–41

Johnstone F D, Abdelmago M S, Harouny A K 1987. Maternal posture in the second stage and fetal acid base status. Br J Obstet Gynaecol 94: 753–757

Jouppila P, Kirkinen P, Koivvla A et al 1983 The influence of maternal oxygen inhalation on human placental and umbilical venous blood flow. Eur J Obstet Gynecol Reprod Biol 16: 151–156

Kelso I M, Parsons R J, Lawrence G F 1978 An assessment of continuous fetal heart rate monitoring in labour. Am J Obstet Gynecol 131: 526

Klink F, Grosspietzsch R, Wlitzing L V et al 1981 Uterine contraction intervals and transcutaneous levels of fetal oxygen pressure. Obstet Gynecol 57: 437–440

Lilja H, Greene K, Karlsson W, Roen K G 1985 ST waveform changes of the fetal ECG during labour: a clinical study. Br J Obstet Gynaecol 92: 611–617

Lilja H, Karlsson K, Lindecrantz K et al 1989 Microprocessor based waveform analysis of the fetal ECG during labour. Int J Gynecol Obstet 30: 109–116

Lofgren O, Jacobson L 1977 Monitoring of transcutaneous pO_2 in the fetus and mother during normal labour. J Perinat Med 6: 252–259

Low J A, Galbraith R S, Muir D W 1983 Intrapartum fetal hypoxia: a study of long term morbidity. Am J Obstet Gynecol 145: 129–134

Maclachlan N A, Spencer J A, Harding K et al 1992 Fetal acidaemia, the CTG and the T/QRS ratio of the fetal ECT in labour. Br J Obstet Gynaecol 99: 26–31

Malcus P, Gudmundsson S, Marshall L et al 1991 Umbilical artery Doppler velocimetry as a labour admission test. Obstet Gynecol 77: 10–16

MacDonald D, Grant A, Sheridan-Pereira M et al 1985 Dublin randomised control trial of antepartum FHR monitoring. Am J Obstet Gynecol 152: 524–539

McNamara H, Chung D C, Lilford R et al 1992 Do fetal pulse oximetry readings at delivery correlate with cord blood oxygenation and acidaemia? Br J Obstet Gynaecol 99: 735–738

Meis P J, Hall M, Marshall J R, Hobel C J 1978 Meconium passage: a new classification of risk assessment during labour. Am J Obstet Gynecol 131: 569–573

Miller F C, Sacks D A, Yeh S et al 1975 The significance of meconium during labour. Am J Obstet Gynecol 122: 573–580

Miyazaki F S, Nevarez F 1985 Saline amnioinfusion for relief of repetitive variable decelerations: a prospective randomised trial. Am J Obstet Gynecol 153: 301–306

Murphy K W, Russell V, Johnson P 1992 Clinical assessment of fetal ECG monitoring in labour. Br J Obstet Gynaecol 99: 32–37

Murray H G 1986 The fetal ECG: current clinical developments in Nottingham. J Perinat Med 14: 399–403

Nelson K B, Ellenberg J H 1984 Obstetric complications and risk factors for cerebral palsy or seizure disorders. J Am Med Assoc 251: 1843–1848

Newbold S, Wheeler T, Clewlow F 1991 Comparison of the T/QRS ratio of the fetal ECG and the FHR during labour and the relation of these variables to the condition at delivery. Br J Obstet Gynaecol 98: 173–178

O'Connor M C, Hytten F E 1979 Measurement of fetal transcutaneous oxygen tension: problem and potential. Br J Obstet Gynaecol 86: 948–953

O'Connor M C, Hytten F E, Zanelli G D 1979 Is the fetus 'scalped' in labour? Lancet ii: 947–948

Okane M, Shigemitsu S, Inaba J et al 1989 Non invasive continuous fetal transcutaneous pO_2 monitoring during labour. J Perinat Med 17: 399–410

Rea P A, Crowe J, Wickramasinghe Y A B D et al 1985 Laser source and detector with signal processor for a NIR medical application. Progress reports on electronics in medicine and biology. IERE, Copeland, pp 209–215

Rolfe P, Burton P J, Crowe J A et al 1982 A fetal scalp mass spectrometer blood gas transducer. J Med Bio Eng Comput 20: 375–382

Rolfe P, Wickramasinghe Y A B D, Thorniley M 1991 The potential of NIRS for detection of fetal cerebral hypoxia. Eur J Obstet Gynecol Reprod Biol 42: S24–28

Rosen K G 1986 Alterations in the fetal ECG as a sign of fetal asphyxia in experimental data with a clinical implementation. J Perinat Med 14: 385–363

Rosen K G, Isaksson O 1976 Alterations in FHR and ECG correlated to glycogen creatine phosphate and ATP levels during graded hypoxia. Biol Neonate 30: 17–24

Rosen K G, Kjellmer I 1975 Change in the fetal heart rate and ECG during hypoxia. Acta Physiol Scand 93: 59–66

Rosen K G, Hokegard W H, Kjellmer I 1976 A study of the relationship between the ECG and haemodynamics of the fetal lamb during asphyxia. Acta Physiol Scand 98: 275–284

Ruth V J, Raivio K O 1988 Perinatal brain damage: predictive value for metabolic acidosis and the Apgar score. Br Med J 297: 24–27

Sasoon D, Castro L, Davis J et al 1990 The biophysical profile in labour. Obstet Gynecol 76: 360–365

Sawers R S 1983 Fetal monitoring during labour. Br Med J 287: 1649–1650

Schmidt S, Gorissen S, Eilers H et al 1991 Animal experiments for the evaluation of laser spectroscopy in the fetus during labour. J Perinat Med 19: 107–113

Shekerloo A, Mendez-Bauerl A, Freese U 1989 Terbutaline for the treatment of acute intrapartum fetal distress. Am J Obstet Gynecol 160: 615–618

Smits T M, Aarnoudse J G, Zijlstra W G 1989 Fetal scalp blood flow as recorded by laser Doppler flowimetry and t_c PO_2 during labour. Early Hum Dev 20: 109–124

Stamm O, Latscha U, Janecek P et al 1974 Kontinuierliche pH messung am kindlichen kopf post partum und sub partu. Z Beburtshilfe Perinatol 178: 368

Sykes G S, Molloy P M, Johnson F et al 1982 Do Apgar scores indicate asphyxia? Lancet i: 494–496

Thaker S B 1987 The efficacy of intrapartum electronic fetal monitoring. Am J Obstet Gynecol 156: 24

Tucker J M, Hauth J C 1990 Intrapartum assessment of fetal wellbeing. Clin Obstet Gynecol 33: 515–553

van der Berg P, Gembruch U, Schmidt S et al 1989 Continuous fetal intrapartum monitoring in SVT by a traumatic measurement of transcutaneous carbon dioxide tension. J Perinat Med 17: 371–374

van der Berg P, Gembruch U, Schmidt S et al 1991 Continuous intrapartum transcutaneous carbon dioxide measurements during fetal arrhythmia. J Perinat Med 19: 81–85

Van Geijn H P, Copray F J, Donkers D K, Bos M H 1991 Diagnosis and management of intrapartum fetal distress. Eur J Obstet Gynecol Reprod Biol 42: S63–S72

Weber T 1979 Continuous measurement of transcutaneous fetal oxygen tension during labour. Br J Obstet Gynaecol 86: 954–958

Wenstrom W D, Parsons M T 1989 The prevention of meconium aspiration in labour using amnioinfusion. Obstet Gynecol 73: 647–657

Westgate J, Harris M, Curnon J S H et al 1992 Randomised trial of CTG alone or with ST waveform analysis for intrapartum monitoring. Lancet 340: 194–198

Wheble A M, Gillmer M D G, Spencer J A D, Sykes G S 1989 Changes in fetal monitoring practice in the U.K.: 1977–1984. Br J Obstet Gynaecol 96: 1140–1147

Zuspan F P, Quilligan E J, Iams T D et al 1979 Predictors of intrapartum fetal distress: the role of electronic fetal monitoring. Am J Obstet Gynecol 35: 287–291

5

Malpractice in obstetrics and gynaecology

R. Doherty   C. E. James

Medical litigation is increasing and claims arising in obstetrics and gynaecology account for the largest proportion settled in hospital practice, reported as 23.7% in a recent survey (James 1991) (Fig. 5.1).

Approximately 30% of damages paid for hospital claims, again the largest proportion for a single specialty, can be attributed to this discipline (Fig. 5.2). In part this reflects the number of claims which relate to alleged 'obstetric' brain damage, but this is a special group for a number of reasons. Firstly, there is no limit of time within which a claim on behalf of a brain-damaged plaintiff can be brought and thus obstetricians may find themselves trying to defend management which took place many years before. Secondly, where negligence can be established, damages are often very large because of the lump-sum nature of most settlements which in addition contain a substantial element to cover the provision of private care for the handicapped child.

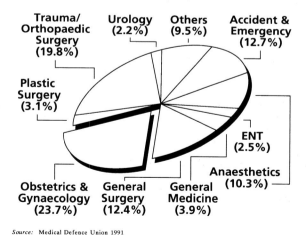

Source: Medical Defence Union 1991

Fig. 5.1 Litigation by hospital specialty in the UK in 1989.

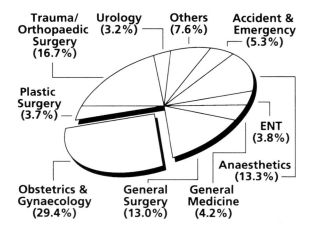

Source: Medical Defence Union 1991

Fig. 5.2.   Indemnity payments made in 1989 in the UK by medical specialty.

Recent changes to the rules governing eligibility for Legal Aid mean that practically all children now qualify and thus can have claims brought on their behalf because assessment of eligibility is independent of parental means. This has resulted in a marked increase in such claims (Capstick & Edwards 1990).

'Obstetric' brain damage litigation does attract considerable publicity and discussion, particularly the debate over the tenuous causal links between perinatal events and subsequent physical and mental development (Nelson 1988, Naeye et al 1989). This is rendered ever more complex because of advances in neonatal care which preserve the lives of many damaged babies who would otherwise have died. However, to concentrate on 'obstetric' brain damage claims gives a distorted view of litigation in the specialty as a whole and diverts attention from other areas where claims could be foreseen more easily and prevented. In this chapter we shall examine the concept of medical negligence and its 'tort'-based system of evaluation; we shall discuss the common causes of litigation in the specialty with reference to the application of risk management principles; we shall outline other areas in which the obstetrician may encounter the law and finally we shall look to the future and possible alternative avenues of compensation and accountability.

COMMON CAUSES OF LITIGATION IN OBSTETRICS

In a recent review of 100 consecutive obstetric claims notified to the Medical Defence Union (MDU) (James 1991) 31% arose from allegations that intrapartum hypoxia resulted in cerebral damage to the neonate, 16% related

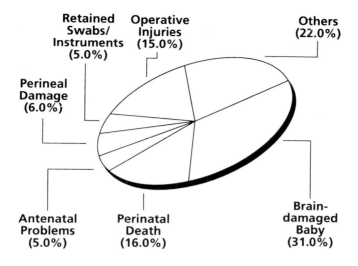

Retained
Swabs/
Instruments
(5.0%)

Operative
Injuries
(15.0%)

Others
(22.0%)

Perineal
Damage
(6.0%)

Antenatal
Problems
(5.0%)

Perinatal
Death
(16.0%)

Brain-
damaged
Baby
(31.0%)

Source: Medical Defence Union 1991

Fig. 5.3. Obstetric claims notified — 100 consecutive cases.

to perinatal death, while 15% followed operative injuries either to mother or baby (Fig. 5.3).

In a similar review of 100 consecutive cases settled, a remarkable 29% involved retained swabs or instruments, 18% operative injuries, and only 9.7% related to hypoxic cerebral damage (Fig. 5.4). The figures, like most statistics in the medicolegal field, are misleading; major claims involving seriously compromised babies are complex and prolonged, while those relating to retained swabs or instruments are incapable of defence and result in rapid settlements. Nevertheless many obstetric claims arise from simple errors and these, in turn, could be prevented by careful adherence to basic principles of risk management.

The antenatal clinic

Many claims arise from failures of communication or resentment, and the antenatal clinic is a fertile field for such claims. Pressure of work in a large clinic may result in a mechanistic 'cattle-market' approach, and prolonged waiting times, lack of privacy, and failure to treat patients with courtesy and respect, may fuel resentment.

History taking

Inadequate or inaccurate history taking may lead to incorrect assumptions on

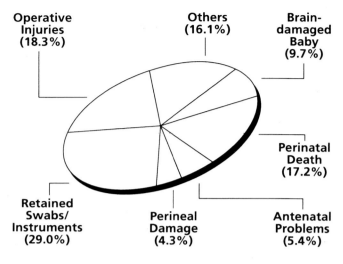

Operative Injuries (18.3%)

Others (16.1%)

Brain-damaged Baby (9.7%)

Perinatal Death (17.2%)

Retained Swabs/ Instruments (29.0%)

Perineal Damage (4.3%)

Antenatal Problems (5.4%)

Source: Medical Defence Union 1991

Fig. 5.4. Obstetric claims settled — 100 consecutive cases.

such basic points as age, parity or menstrual history; if such mistakes are prolonged throughout the antenatal period, decision making on the method of delivery based on such inaccuracies may lead to major errors. Language difficulties often inhibit communication in areas with a large multi-ethnic population.

Identification of high-risk pregnancy

Divided views remain on the merits of routine regular antenatal care, but failure to identify high-risk pregnancy, leading to inadequate monitoring, non-referral for specialist advice, and failure to establish a proper plan for the management of labour, may lead to major errors and to claims.

Shared care

Where antenatal care is shared between general practitioner (GP) and hospital, good communication is essential. Information contained in GP and hospital clinical records should be freely available to parties and, if a cooperation card is used, this should be accurately and fully completed. A GP concerned at any adverse factor should have ready access to consultant opinion.

Record keeping

The importance of full and accurate records must be stressed. The standard continues to be poor and lack of continuity of care, often said to be inevitable in large maternity hospitals, coupled with inadequate records, may lead to important information being lost. Hospitals, health authorities and trusts have a duty to ensure that antenatal records are carefully stored and easily available for antenatal clinics, and also to ensure that results of investigations are checked on receipt in case urgent action is needed, and then filed in the correct records.

Ultrasound and amniocentesis

Careful identification of the patient at risk, and awareness of the need in high-risk pregnancy for ultrasound or amniocentesis to be carried out where facilities are available, are essential to good antenatal care. An increasing number of claims relate to failure to identify growth retardation in utero, and failure to detect babies with Down's syndrome by amniocentesis.

Consultant supervision

Too many patients, booked for hospital delivery under consultant care, are never seen by a consultant during the antenatal period. Statements of claim, in obstetric cases, often put heavy emphasis on this fact. There is a general and understandable expectation that a patient referred to hospital for consultant care will obtain it.

Patients' requests and anxieties

A dismissive or paternalistic approach to patients' concerns is a common cause of resentment when an obstetric accident has occurred. There are, of course, over-demanding and obsessive patients who take up a disproportionate amount of time, but the well-worn adage 'listen to the patient, she knows when things are going wrong' should not be forgotten. Patients' preference for the conduct of their labours should be noted; if it is felt that patients' wishes cannot be accommodated, this should be explained and an alternative referral made if necessary.

The labour ward

Problems arising in the labour ward which commonly give rise to claims usually result either from failures of communication or of supervision. This is particularly so when a team approach is used. It is only too easy, in a busy unit, for an outgoing team to omit to pass on to its successors early warning of abnormalities in a cardiotocographic (CTG) trace.

An incoming team may have other duties; claims have arisen when a team, starting work at lunch-time, has an afternoon commitment to an antenatal clinic, and a patient, fully dilated at change-over time, is allowed to remain too long in the second stage before medical help is summoned.

CTG Traces

CTG traces are only as valuable as those who interpret them. In a recent risk management survey carried out by the MDU, it was found that neither midwives nor senior house officers (SHOs) received any formal training in the interpretation of CTGs; too much reliance was placed on the opinion of a registrar, who was often not easily available. All traces should be labelled accurately, timed, and carefully retained in the clinical records; absence of a relevant CTG trace induces suspicion in the minds of lawyers, and makes successful defence of allegations of inadequate monitoring difficult to rebut.

Records

General guidance again applies, but labour records are critically important in ensuring continuity of care and also in proving that supervision was adequate. Partograms, if used, must be completed accurately, and all entries should be correctly dated and timed, and signed in an identifiable way by the author.

Protocols

Clear protocols should be available to nursing and medical staff on procedures to be carried out, and the calling of medical aid. Experienced midwives should not hesitate to contact a senior member of the medical team directly in appropriate circumstances.

Protocols should not be too proscriptive, but should give general guidelines. It is important that outdated protocols should be retained, with a note made of the date of introduction of the revised protocol.

Consultant supervision

While proper delegation of duties to junior medical staff, properly trained, may be appropriate, consultants bear the ultimate responsibility for events in their units and must make themselves available, if called. Routine labour ward rounds pay great dividends, not only to peace of mind but also to a proper understanding of what is going on in the unit.

Instrumental and breech deliveries

Instrumental and breech deliveries should only be carried out by medical staff competent in the procedures. Early training and supervision is essential.

Rotational forceps deliveries are not for the inexperienced, unless very closely supervised.

Availability of expert anaesthetic and paediatric staff

It is essential to modern-day obstetrics that expert anaesthetic and paediatric staff are available, particularly where delivery may be complex, as in twins, breech and instrumental deliveries. Problems of understaffing and in the provision of services to isolated or outlying units do not provide adequate grounds for defence when delay in delivery or resuscitation leads to hypoxic brain damage.

Caesarean section

It is only too easy for a plaintiff to argue that, where an obstetric accident has occurred, earlier resort to Caesarean section would have prevented the outcome. Sources of delay which commonly result in claims include late decision making, non-availability of theatres, medical staff or transport facilities. Damage to mother or baby during Caesarean section is often seen as negligent despite operative difficulties. It is vital that damage be identified and quickly rectified, and that full and sympathetic explanations are given to the patient, together with proper apologies where appropriate.

The postnatal period

Common pitfalls are:

1. Failure to arrange rubella immunization for a seronegative mother
2. Failure to give Anti-D immune globulin where appropriate
3. Failure to arrange or monitor Guthrie tests and screening tests for hypothyroidism on the baby
4. Retained swabs.

Earlier discharge from hospital means that the optimum time for Guthrie testing arises after the infant has gone home. In this circumstance, failures of communication between hospital, GPs and community midwives increase the potential for error. Secondary postpartum haemorrhage arising after discharge and requiring readmission for curettage brings allegations of inadequate postnatal supervision. It is usually assumed that this can be foreseen and prevented. Although such cases can be defended, adequate defence is easier when it can be shown that uterine involution was carefully monitored. The examination for discharge is not a meaningless ritual and should be recorded carefully.

COMMON PROBLEMS IN GYNAECOLOGY

Claims arising from gynaecological practice are, on the whole, less expensive to meet than those arising from obstetric practice, but the consequences of a gynaecological mishap can be just as devastating for the patient and as stressful and time-consuming for the doctors involved.

Failure to obtain informed consent

When consent is sought for a gynaecological procedure, as in any other situation, the patient must be fully aware of the nature of the procedure to be carried out, and its material risks and side-effects. There is a popular misconception that where an operation results in sterilization, consent of the spouse must be obtained. This is not so, but it is good practice where a stable relationship exists for both partners to be counselled so that they understand fully the implications.

Sterilizations

The risk of failure of the operation to achieve its purpose is a material risk and one of which the patient must be made aware. The consent form or the clinical record must contain a detailed note that this warning has been given. Counselling should also be given on alternative methods of contraception.

Hysterectomy

Patients are sometimes unaware that hysterectomy inevitably results in sterility, or that vaginal function can be fully maintained after the operation. Explanations given should be in simple terms, with no assumption made that the patient has a knowledge of anatomy.

Where a salpingo-oophorectomy is to be part of the operation, this should be fully explained and specific consent obtained. Failure to warn of the need for salpingo-oophorectomy, or failure to heed the patient's wishes in this regard, frequently results in claims that an unnecessary castrating operation has been carried out. It can be, at least, imprudent to embark on myomectomy without obtaining consent for hysterectomy should the need arise.

Vaginal hysterectomy, particularly if accompanied by a vaginal repair, requires careful counselling. If stress incontinence is treated by colporrhaphy, the possible need for a repeat operation should be explained since patients' expectation of complete cure at the first attempt are high.

Ectopic pregnancy

Claims are sometimes made that delayed diagnosis of tubal pregnancy results in a salpingo-oophorectomy, with consequent effects on fertility, which could have been avoided had the condition been detected earlier. In acute cases it may seldom be possible to give adequate preoperative counselling, but the treatment given and its sequelae should be fully explained during the postoperative period.

Operative injuries

Operative injuries may be unavoidable in gynaecological surgery, but should be fully explained to the patient. Essential to a successful defence in such cases are early recognition and correction, and keeping the patient fully informed and reassured. To damage a ureter during hysterectomy is not, of itself, necessarily negligent; negligence may arise if the injury is not identified or if it is dealt with incorrectly.

Swabs and instruments

Swabs and instruments continue, with depressing frequency, to be retained during obstetric and gynaecological operations. Sound technique and correct operating theatre procedures are necessary.

Laparoscopy

Laparoscopy is not a simple procedure to be delegated to inexperienced juniors; even in the most expert hands there are risks of damage to intra-abdominal or retroperitoneal structures. There is a need to consider the possibility of pre-existing pregnancy when carrying out tubal ligation either by laparoscopy or by open techniques.

Perforation of the uterus

Perforation of the uterus during curettage is not uncommon, and in the pregnant or puerperal uterus, or in the presence of malignancy, may form a natural hazard of the operation, and accidental perforation may be defensible. Careful monitoring after perforation and, if necessary, operative intervention is essential.

Endometrial ablation

A number of claims have already been made relating to this treatment; almost all relate to perforation of the uterus, or injury to the pelvic structures.

THE OBSTETRICIAN AS A WITNESS

An obstetrician may find himself as witness in a number of situations, but primarily these will be as a professional witness to fact on behalf of one of his patients or at an inquest. He may also appear before the General Medical Council (GMC), as a defendant in a civil claim or a criminal action brought either by or on behalf of one of his patients, or as an 'expert' giving his opinion for either plaintiff or defendant in a case in which he has no personal involvement. In each situation it is as well for the obstetrician to be aware of what is expected.

As a professional witness to fact the clinician may be approached by a coroner's officer (acting on behalf of the coroner), the police, or solicitors for a report on aspects of a patient's care. Only the coroner has statutory powers to request such information, and in other circumstances a doctor must ensure that the proper consent has been obtained from the patient or, if deceased, the patient's personal representative. Medical practitioners should bear in mind that their actions may be criticized if they are required to give evidence at an inquest, and they are advised to seek medicolegal advice from their health authority or defence organization before submitting a report when they believe the circumstances could be contentious.

Civil actions

In these days of increasing litigation an obstetrician is likely to find himself the subject of a possible civil claim from one of his patients at least once if not more during his professional life-time (Saunders 1992, Malkasian 1991). The incident giving rise to such litigation is often one which causes considerable disquiet at the time, and defence organizations are frequently asked what it is appropriate to tell the patient in these circumstances. The MDU has published its view (Allsopp 1986) that the patient is entitled to a full and frank explanation of events, together with an expression of sympathy for whatever mishap has occurred. Speculation on the facts, attribution of blame and a formal admission of liability should, however, be avoided.

It is often helpful in a case where litigation seems likely for the doctor to prepare an account of events as soon as possible, whilst the patient's management is fresh in his mind. This report should identify all the key personnel involved, with full names if possible, and should be filed confidentially, separately from the case records. This is an extension of the system of untoward incident reporting which is a major component of any 'risk management' programme, now increasingly being introduced enthusiastically into many UK obstetric and gynaecological departments.

Once litigation has been notified, the obstetrician will be asked to prepare a detailed report for his health authority or medical defence organization in order to assist in the assessment of allegations which the patient has put forward. It is useful for this to be submitted in two parts: a factual account of personal involvement in the case, and a covering letter in which interpretative comments, opinions or criticisms can be expressed on the matter generally. This report should not be filed in the patient's case notes as it is a document prepared in response to the litigation process and therefore should not form part of the records to be disclosed.

Expert witness

Clearly, for the patient to bring her case she needs to be assisted not only by lawyers but by a doctor who will advise on the strengths and weaknesses of her claim — the 'plaintiff's expert'. In these days of increasing litigation many obstetricians are being asked to act in this capacity, as well as to report for defendant health authorities, trusts and the medical defence organizations. This work is time consuming but should be given serious consideration by obstetricians of suitable experience, since an objective and informed report at an early stage is beneficial to both professional colleagues and patients, as well as being interesting and educational for the 'expert'. When embarking on the preparation of expert reports the obstetrician would be advised to follow the guidelines, which for simplicity are set out in Table 5.1.

When a patient resorts to law it is the clinicians, not the lawyers, who set the standards by which the patient's care is judged, and this underlines the importance of expert witnesses being recruited among those obstetricians who are or who have recently been engaged in active practice, and whose experience is relevant and contemporary to the events in question.

Table 5.1   Preparation of expert reports

1. When first approached seek advice on the format of reports from experienced colleagues or a medical defence organization
2. Always ensure you have all the relevant notes, legal documents etc. before expressing a view, and list the material on which your report is based in its introduction
3. Judge the claim in accordance with the definition of medical neligence and with the standard of care relevant to the date of events
4. Differentiate the harm, if any, caused by the medical negligence, from that which may have been expected in any event
5. Support opinions by reference to contemporary authoritative texts, papers or official guidelines
6. Avoid gratuitous criticism of colleagues
7. If asked to comment on the patient's current condition and prognosis do not confuse this with a view on liability, which should be given separately
8. Be prepared to endorse the views you have expressed publicly and under cross-examination in court if necessary

Criminal prosecution/General Medical Council

An obstetrician may find himself accountable not only in civil cases but also to the criminal courts, his professional registration body and his employing health authority or trust. Charges of manslaughter and murder have recently been brought against doctors (Dyer 1991, Brahams 1992) which have been successful, at least in the court of first instance.

In addition, early in 1992 the GMC proposed an extension of its role such that it would be enabled to investigate cases where a doctor's general pattern of practice was so poor as to put patients at risk. This proposal was accepted at the end of 1992 and parliamentary time is now being sought for a Bill to make the necessary amendments to the 1983 Medical Act to allow the new procedure to commence as soon as possible. A new committee of the GMC would be set up to investigate cases where there is a suggestion of a serious deficiency in a doctor's performance. This would add a further form of accountability to the increasingly used hospital complaints and disciplinary procedures.

RECENT LEGAL CHANGES

In November 1990 the law governing abortion in Britain was fundamentally altered by the passage of the Human Fertilization and Embryology Act 1990. Its provisions, like those of the Abortion Act 1967, do not apply to Northern Ireland, nor has the situation changed in the Republic of Ireland (Orr 1990), although a referendum on the subject was held at the end of 1992.

In order to understand the British changes a brief historical resumé is required. The basic statute governing abortion remains the Offences Against the Person Act 1861, and abortions are only lawful as a result of exceptions to that Act. In 1929 a further statute — the Infant Life Preservation Act — was introduced to protect the child who was still in utero but was capable of being born alive, since the common law of murder can apply once the baby has been fully expelled from its mother's body. The Abortion Act 1967 did not alter the protection offered to a child under the 1929 Act — it merely created a defence to prosecution, provided termination was performed within its four stipulated clauses. These referred to risk to the physical or mental health of the mother or existing children, the mother's life and the possibility of serious mental or physical handicap in the unborn child.

For many years, 28 weeks was accepted as the gestation after which a baby was 'capable of being born alive' and was reflected in many definitions and statutory obligations associated with the registration of births and deaths.

Legal precedent caught up with neonatal advances in 1990 in the judgement of Mr Justice Brooke in *Rance* v. *Mid-Downs Health Authority and Storr* (Brahams 1990), when the Infant Life Preservation Act 1929 was interpreted as protecting every fetus able to sustain life independent of its mother. Although a lower limit of gestation was not specified the logic of this decision would have been to protect the fetus from 23 or 24 weeks onwards.

Some changes in the amended law on abortion also reflect the decreasing age of fetal viability. The relevant section of the Human Fertilization and Embryology Act 1990 which came into force in April 1991 now allows termination of pregnancy on the grounds of risk to the mental or physical health of the mother or her existing children only up to a specifically stated gestation of *24* weeks. The statutory definition of stillbirth in Great Britain and Northern Ireland has been similarly reduced from 28 to 24 weeks as of October 1992.

The vast majority of late terminations of pregnancy are not performed for so-called 'social' indications but because of suspected serious fetal abnormalities. No sooner had Mr Justice Brooke's judgement (see above) given some guidance to those involved in antenatal diagnosis, than it became redundant by a further provision of the Human Fertilization and Embryology Act 1990 which allows termination to be performed *without limit of time* (by virtue of a repeal in the Infant Life Preservation Act 1929), where continuation of the pregnancy may result in grave permanent harm to the health of the mother, where there is risk to her life or where there is substantial risk of severe fetal handicap.

Thus, theoretically at least, termination of pregnancy is now permitted in such circumstances up to and including term, but clearly at such an advanced gestation the baby would be capable of being born alive by any definition. The repeal of the Infant Life Preservation Act 1929 in these cases protects the obstetrician only as far as the unborn child is concerned. If an attempted termination results in a live birth with subsequent death or handicap he may become involved in both civil and criminal proceedings.

Before leaving the subject of abortion mention should be made of selective reduction of pregnancy — a solution to the 'overladen lifeboat' described so appositely in Orr (1990). The legality of this procedure has now been clarified in that it may now be performed within the defined criteria applicable to other terminations and subject to statutory notification.

Notwithstanding the above comments, the casual observer could be forgiven for failing to make any connection between the Human Fertilization and Embryology Act 1990 and abortion; the relevant sections were added as the Bill went through Parliament and the Act's primary purpose was to make statutory provision for the licensing of certain types of assisted conception and to control and supervise research involving human embryos. This function had previously been undertaken on a non-statutory basis by the Voluntary Licensing Authority (VLA).

Apparently intentionally, the confidentiality provisions of the Act (introduced in August 1991) were very restrictive and prevented a licensed practitioner from disclosing information about his patient in connection with the provision of fertility treatment services. Effectively this prevented the direct exchange of information with GPs and other non-licensed doctors. It also deprived the licensed doctor of his ability to defend himself should litigation or complaint arise. These problems have now largely been resolved following the introduction, in July 1992, of the Human Fertilization and Embryology (Disclosure of Information) Act.

It could fairly be said, however that neither the abortion nor the infertility sections of the Human Fertilization and Embryology Act 1990 have defined parameters that the practising obstetrician and gynaecologist may have wished. Perhaps this is inevitable when the law tries to deal with emotive ethical issues.

THE FUTURE

When a patient complains about her treatment the present tort-based system of litigation deals primarily with only one aspect, namely financial compensation. The patient herself may require satisfaction on a wider front, with deterrence, punishment and explanation all being additional objectives. Those interested in more detailed analysis of these complex interactions and their relation to litigation and complaints will find them discussed informatively by Whelan (1988). Suffice to say that effective systems to redress the harm suffered by victims of medical accidents need to take into account both compensation and accountability. The alternatives to the established tort system which have already been discussed, such as 'no fault' compensation and arbitration, do not deal with the latter. Neither does the present tort system hold the doctor accountable: the more obviously negligent a patient's treatment, the more likely there is to be a settlement out of court.

That the patient wants accountability cannot be denied. In New Zealand, a country which has operated a type of 'no fault' compensation since 1974, there has been a 2000% increase in complaints to the Medical Practitioners Disciplinary Council, the local equivalent of the UK's GMC, since the scheme was inaugurated (James 1992).

The GMC's increased interest in complaints concerning clinical matters and its proposed performance review procedure are an indication of its response to public pressure and dissatisfaction, as is the apparent increase in complaints, inquiries, disciplinary investigations and criminal proceedings brought to the attention of the medical defence organizations.

Litigation and complaints are a particular problem to the obstetrician, and concern has been expressed that this is leading to defensive practices and diminished recruitment to the specialty. With regard to the former a recent survey in the UK indicated that tests deemed to be inaccurate may nevertheless be used in clinical practice because some obstetricians fear litigation (Ennis et al 1991). In a study undertaken by the Royal College of Obstetricians and Gynaecologists (RCOG) (Saunders 1992) responses suggested that medicolegal problems played a less important role in career choice. The Chief Medical Officer for England and Wales in his William Power lecture to the Royal College of Midwives in 1990 was of the view that recruitment would be affected, and personal emotional trauma seemed an important influence on doctors throughout their training period. On the other hand, fear of litigation does seem to have influenced the retention within the specialty of practising obstetricians. Both an RCOG survey quoted by Saunders (1992) and the 1990 survey of American obstetricians (Malkasian 1991) indicate that obstetricians are now favouring early retirement, and in the USA over 12% have ceased obstetric practice because of the malpractice risk.

CONCLUSION

Obstetrics and gynaecology remains a medicolegal minefield, but with careful clinical management, audit and application of risk management principles, involvement in litigation should be minimized. This chapter has highlighted some common problems, explained some recent legal changes and looked into the future. It is hoped it will assist the beleaguered practitioner to avoid the obvious dangers and pitfalls.

KEY POINTS FOR CLINICAL PRACTICE

To avoid medical accidents and to avoid allegations of malpractice, it is necessary to observe certain key points in clinical practice, and no apology is made for stressing these:

1. *Conscientious practice.* No doctor deliberately sets out to practise negligently, but inattention to detail, a laissez faire attitude and the taking of clinical short cuts lead almost inevitably to allegations of negligence.

2. *Good communication* between doctor and patient, not always easy for either party, is essential. This is particularly so when a medical accident has occurred.

3. *Careful records.* The need for these cannot be over-stressed. Consultants have a duty to ensure that records kept by their juniors are full, accurate and contemporaneous; an equal duty falls on the consultant to maintain good records whether in public or private practice.

4. *Informed consent.* It is essential that patients should give fully informed consent to all treatment.

5. *Proper delegation.* Only delegate to others tasks which they are fully competent to carry out.

6. *Risk management.* Many claims can be prevented by attention to risk management principles. A proper awareness of what may lead to claims, and identification of risk areas within a unit, together with a system of adverse incident reporting, will permit corrective action. Consultants have a duty to identify and draw attention to deficiencies in resources or staffing which may adversely affect patient care.

REFERENCES

Allsopp K M 1986 Saying sorry. J Medical Defence Union 2:2:2
Brahams D 1990 Judicial warning on very late abortions. Lancet i: 464
Brahams D 1992 Euthanasia: doctor convicted of attempted murder. Lancet 340: 782–378
Capstick J B, Edwards P J 1990 Trends in obstetric malpractice claims. Lancet 336: 931–932
Dyer C 1991 Doctors convicted of manslaughter: Br Med J 303: 1157

Ennis M, Clark A, Grudzinkas J G 1991 Changes in obstetric practice in response to fear of litigation in the British Isles. Lancet 338: 616–618

James C E 1991 Risk management in obstetrics and gynaecology. J Medical Defence Union 2: 36–38

James C 1992 Professional accountability in New Zealand 1974–1991: doctor, patient and advocate: compensation and accountability: keeping the balance.In: Wall J (ed) Proceedings of a Medical Defence Union Conference: May 1991. Mercury Books, London, pp 7–25

Malkasian G D 1991. Professional liability and the delivery of obstetrical care. Am Coll Surg Bull 76: 6–12, 37

Naeye R L, Peters E C, Bartholomew M, Landis R L 1989 Origins of cerebral palsy. Am J Dis Child 143: 1154–1161

Nelson K 1988 What proportion of cerebral palsy is related to birth asphyxia? J. Pediatr 112: 572–574

Orr C 1990 Medicolegal aspects of obstetric and gynaecological practice. In: Bonnar J (ed) Recent advances in obstetrics and gynaecology 16. Churchill Livingstone, Edinburgh, pp 111–123

Saunders P 1992 Recruitment in obstetrics and gynaecology. RCOG sets initiatives. Br J Obstet Gynaecol 99: 538–546

Whelan C J 1988 Litigation and complaints procedures, objectives, effectiveness and alternatives. J Med Ethics 14: 70–76

Fertility

6

Update on male infertility

H. W. G. Baker   E. J. Keogh

For some infertile men the treatment we provide in the late twentieth century differs very little from that offered by Galen in AD 160. Their disorder is not understood and the treatment has scarce scientific support. Conversely, some causes of infertility have been defined precisely at an electron microscopic and molecular biology level and for these treatment is specific, simple and gratifying. The compulsion by the doctor to do something, indeed anything, to overcome the couple's distress is as great as ever.

Success in the arena of assisted reproductive technology has been spectacular for those having donor insemination, and less so with in vitro fertilization (IVF) and gamete intrafallopian tube transfer (GIFT). Most advances have occurred this century — especially IVF.

Infertility is the failure to produce a pregnancy within 12 months of trying. Subfertility implies a less severe impairment of fertility in which there is no identifiable major impediment such as azoospermia (Table 6.1). Fifty per cent of normal couples conceive within 5 months, and 85% within 12 months. Second pregnancies occur sooner, 50% within 2 months. In Western countries 15% of couples are infertile and 24% of UK women experience infertility at some stage in their lives (Greenhall & Vessey 1990). In roughly half the husband has reduced fertility. However, 25% of women whose husbands were azoospermic and 50% of women whose husbands had normal semen had abnormalities such as anovulation or damaged fallopian tubes. The phenomenon of both partners contributing to infertility is also illustrated by a WHO study in which 26.5% of 8500 couples had both male and female factors operating to reduce the likelihood of conception (Comhaire et al 1987). Donor insemination is more successful in partners of azoospermic men than partners of oligospermic ($<20 \times 10^6$/ml) men. When men with

Table 6.1 Definitions of male infertility

Azoospermia — no sperm in the ejaculate
Oligospermia — $<20 \times 10^6$ sperm/ml
Asthenozoospermia — $<50\%$ of sperm with forward motility or $<25\%$ with rapid linear motility
Teratozoospermia — $<30\%$ sperm with normal morphology

Kallmann's syndrome (azoospermia, low follicle stimulating hormone (FSH) and luteinizing hormone (LH)) are given exogenous FSH and LH, their wives sometimes conceive after only small increments in sperm concentrations. Thus the wives of men with moderately low counts are more likely to be contributing to the problem, by ovulatory or tubal disorders or unexplained mechanisms.

AETIOLOGY

Most infertile men cannot be given a precise explanation of the pathology and prognosis of their disorder. Nonetheless Table 6.2 demonstrates a systematic approach to male infertility. An alternative approach in Table 6.3 (Baker et al 1986) shows the categories of treatable male infertility and the frequency of each group. After excluding other disorders most have subnormal or abnormal sperm production for which we cannot offer an accurate diagnosis. Currently treatment regimens remain controversial or are the subject of incomplete therapeutic trials.

HISTORY

It is preferable but not always possible to interview both partners simultaneously. Their initial reaction to the interview is not invariably positive.

Table 6.2   Causes of male infertility

A. SPERM PRODUCTION
a   Stimulation of testis reduced
    Hypothalamic — GnRH deficiency
    Pituitary — gonadotrophin (FSH and LH) deficiency; tumour, hypophysectomy
    testosterone therapy (athletes)
b   Stimulation of testis increased
    unresponsive to elevated FSH and LH — previous cryptorchidism, torsion, mumps in
    adulthood, cytotoxics for cancer, Klinefelter's syndrome
c   Normal stimulation of testis unresponsive to normal FSH and LH — idiopathic
    hypospermatogenesis

B   SPERM DELIVERY
Congenital absence of efferent ducts, obstruction of epididymis, infection, congenital absence
of vas, inspissated mucus (Young's syndrome), coital abnormalities

C   IMMOTILE SPERM
Immotile cilia syndrome — electron microscopic morphology abnormal
Accessory gland infection — morphology normal
Sperm transport defects — sperm autoimmunity

D   FUTURE CLASSIFICATIONS MAY INCLUDE:
Sperm acrosomal defects
Zona binding defects
Zona penetration defects
Oolemma fusion defects
Pronucleus formation defects

Table 6.3 Treatability of male infertility

A UNTREATABLE STERILITY	12.8%
Primary seminiferous tubule failure	12.8%
B TREATABLE CONDITIONS	12.1%
Gonadotrophin deficiency	0.6%
Obstructive azoospermia	5.0%
Sperm autoimmunity	6.0%
Disorders of sexual function	0.5%
Reversible toxic effects	0.02%
C UNTREATABLE SUBFERTILITY	75%
Oligospermia	38%
Asthenospermia, teratospermia	37%

Negative, hostile or disinterested men may feel coerced by their wives. Such reactions and dynamics of the couples are most apparent in the first 10 minutes of the interview. Time must be invested in establishing rapport if one hopes subsequently to obtain semen, blood and postcoital samples. If there are potentially divisive matters unearthed during history taking, such as pregnancies from another man or VD, it may be teased out over several interviews, some of which may need to be with only one member of the couple.

Duration of infertility

If the couple are young and not obviously sterile it is reasonable to allow a year of unprotected intercourse before becoming concerned about infertility. However, if the woman is over 35 years of age or if there are known impediments to their fertility (e.g. previous mumps or cryptorchidism) investigations can be initiated earlier. In this context a normal or near-normal semen analysis is reassuring. Beyond 35 years amniocentesis or chorionic villous biopsy appears to be mandatory, adding another threat to the unborn which may be avoided by initiating investigations earlier for older couples.

Family history

Idiopathic oligospermia tends to run in families, as does Young's syndrome. Kallmann's syndrome and dystrophia myotonica are genetically determined. Sperm autoimmunity tends to accompany organ-specific autoimmune disease of the thyroid and gastric parietal cells. Bilateral congenital absence of the vas deferens is frequently (50–60%) associated with heterozygosity for the common cystic fibrosis gene (delta F 508).

Adequacy and timing of intercourse

The man must appreciate the need for depositing the sperm deep in the vagina during intercourse. This ought to coincide with ovulation, which most women recognize by increased mucous discharge. By virtue of occult hostility, abhorrence of pregnancy, low libido, itinerant occupations or shiftwork, intercourse for some couples is a monthly event, or at best every two weeks. Rarely, couples will participate in invasive investigations for infertility over several years before confessing to impotence or other hidden agendas whereby they sabotage their management. Attempts to predetermine sex by having intercourse early or late relative to ovulation may compromise the fertility of those who have minor problems. A basic lesson with take-home illustrations on ovulation and coitus enables the doctor to evaluate their comprehension and attend to gaps in their knowledge. Patient-inspired books and videos on these topics are also useful.

Childhood and pubertal development

Prenatal exposure to diethylstilboestrol may cause epididymal malformations, undescended testes and oligospermia. Epispadias, hypospadias, urethral valves, inguinal hernias, hydroceles, major urogenital malformations and their surgical treatment may impair fertility. Delayed puberty raises the possibility of Kallmann's syndrome, or other hypothalamic and/or pituitary disorders. Conversely, accelerated puberty culminating in short stature suggests congenital adrenal hyperplasia.

General health

Any illness can reduce sperm production and libido. Fever, irrespective of cause, may reduce sperm output for several months. The onset of diabetes mellitus may be accompanied by neuropathy leading to impotence and retrograde ejaculation. Renal failure is complicated; there are metabolic factors, cytotoxic drugs, zinc deficiency, damage to vasa and diversion of the penile blood supply to the transplanted kidney. Hepatic dysfunction presents a similar pattern of decompensation, but despite these metabolic insults sperm production and fertility are often normal. In this context, alcohol and recreational drug abuse must be severe to impair fertility (Oldereid et al 1989). Paraplegia and quadriplegia result in 'paralytic obstructive azoospermia' and anejaculation.

Respiratory disease

Chronic sinusitis, bronchiectasis and obstruction of the epididymides by inspissated mucus are hallmarks of Young's syndrome. The history is more informative than physical examination. Bronchiectasis also occurs with immotile cilia and situs inversus may exist. Males with cystic fibrosis usually have bilateral congenital absence of the vasa.

Undescended testes

In Melbourne, 7.7% of infertile men gave a history of maldescent. A follow-up study of men operated upon for undescended testes conducted in Perth (Australia) revealed azoospermia in most who had bilateral maldescent as children and severe oligospermia in 75% of those operated upon for unilateral maldescent. However, orchidopexy is not the complete answer. Given that 1% of boys at 1 year of age have this disorder it is one of the potentially remediable lesions causing infertility. The possibility exists that the testis is innately abnormal and, irrespective of treatment, scrotal position etc, will be unable to produce adequate sperm.

Testicular pain and swelling

Often this occurs 10–15 years prior to the problem of infertility and the details are sketchy. Nonetheless, torsion, orchitis, epididymitis or epididymo-orchitis may be manifest as swelling followed by atrophy. Delay in treating venereal infections may be evident on discovery of a swollen irregular epididymis. Frequently the patients are unaware of these abnormalities, or indeed of the preceding infection. Men with prostatic infection may have post-ejaculatory burning at the tip of the penis and prostatic tenderness on examination. Torsion surgery may have been delayed, resulting in testicular atrophy, and the anchoring suture in the contralateral testis may inadvertently damage and obstruct the epididymis.

Iatrogenic

Pelvic and inguinal surgery may compromise the blood supply of the vasa or testes. Renal transplantation, hydrocele, epididymal cyst or varicocele surgery may inadvertently lead to reduced fertility. Chemotherapy and X-ray therapy for testicular tumours, leukaemia or lymphoma deplete the germinal epithelium, leaving behind the supporting Sertoli cells. Histologically it is known as the Sertoli cell only syndrome and is usually irreversible. By contrast, sulphasalazine (Wu et al 1989) for ulcerative colitis induces a reversible reduction of spermatogenesis. Athletes who use enormous doses of androgens and anabolic agents may have a return to normal fertility once they stop the drugs. Less commonly, oestrogen, glucocorticoids, cimetidine, spironolactone, nitrofurantoin, hypotensive agents and psychotropic drugs in large doses may cause infertility.

Occupation and lifestyle

Foundry workers, drivers (especially if obese), spa and sauna devotees may unwittingly heat the testes and jeopardize sperm production. Occupational exposure to nematocides, organophosphates, oestrogen, benzene, zinc, lead, cadmium and mercury are recognized and avoided by employers and most employees alike nowadays (Henderson et al 1986).

PHYSICAL EXAMINATION

During a complete physical examination particular attention is paid to the following issues. The signs of masculinization vary according to ethnic group, occupation, parental traits etc. Change is important. If a Chinese man loses body hair and shaves less often, it is probably clinically significant, whereas similar changes may go unnoticed in a southern Italian. Delayed epiphyseal fusion in Asians and Caucasians is evident if the arm span exceeds height by 5 cm. This indicates some delay in the pubertal onset of androgen secretion. Gynaecomastia is uncommon but indicates a significant surplus of oestrogen relative to androgen. Such men may, have small and/or soft testes. Examination of the penile shaft may reveal Peyronie's disease (as a cause of impotence) or meatal anomalies.

Scrotum and its contents

Scrotal scars, often forgotten by the patient, may indicate previous trauma or surgery. Skin abnormalities may reduce heat loss from the testes, which are normally 4–5°C below body core temperature. The testicular position is important in view of the poor fertility associated with testes lying outside the scrotum. Testicular volume is most conveniently measured with the Prader orchidometer — a series of plastic ellipsoids from 1 to 25 ml which are held adjacent to the testis. Other methods using callipers or tapes will suffice. Generally, over 20 ml is normal; the left testis is often slightly smaller. The testis is comprised, in the main (90%), of sperm-producing tissue; it is not surprising therefore that size is correlated with number of sperm in the ejaculate. Furthermore, bigger men have larger testes.

Tenderness may persist for many years after mumps orchitis; conversely, reduced testicular sensation may reflect autonomic neuropathy, chronic inflammation or neoplasia. The testes may be rotated on their long axes so that the epididymis lies anterior, or they may lie horizontally. This does not seem to affect fertility adversely.

Varicoceles

Varicoceles are usually confined to the left side and are graded as follows: (1) cough impulse only (observed in spermatic cord held between the index finger and thumb while patient is supine): (2) palpable enlarged veins (these will be missed if the patient does not do the Valsalva manoeuvre in the standing position); (3) visible enlarged veins.

Epididymis

The head of the epididymis is gently palpated; this structure is often tender despite a negative history of infection. If there is a blockage at the junction of the middle and upper thirds it is usually reflected in doubling or trebling of its size, made all the more conspicuous by the relative atrophy of the body and tail of the epididymis. The size of the epididymis is governed by androgen secretion, some of which is transported via rete testis fluid. Small testes associated with normal-sized epididymides suggests postpubertal atrophy. By contrast, small epididymides and testes suggest abnormal puberty, e.g. Kallman's syndrome. Irregularities and thickening of the epididymides suggest chronic infection (e.g. gonorrhoea) leading to obstruction. Vasectomized men may have thickened, irregular epididymides. Anatomical variants such as a cyst of Morgagni may cause confusion about the head of the epididymis but are irrelevant.

Vas deferens

This duct is readily palpated in the spermatic cord. It is smooth, about 3 mm in diameter, firm and non-tender. Typically, male genital tuberculosis is manifest as beading and rigidity of the vas and epididymis. The vas may be congenitally absent; usually the seminal vesicles are also absent, reflecting their common embryological origin. Low seminal plasma fructose confirms this diagnosis.

LABORATORY TESTS

Semen analysis

We provide a suitable room adjacent to the laboratory and the laboratory staff arrange for the on-site collection of semen. A sterile transparent, plastic jar (4.5 cm diameter, 5 cm deep) is weighed before collection, and the ejaculate volume is then measured by the total weight minus the tare. Written instructions specify a 3-day abstinence prior to collection and avoidance of any petroleum-based creams or soap which may reduce sperm motility. Men who can only produce ejaculates during intercourse may need to use coitus interruptus or non-toxic condoms. Latex inhibits sperm motility, as do the lubricants and additives used in condom manufacture. If these measures fail the postcoital sampling of semen from the vagina may suffice. For men who cannot ejaculate normally non-toxic condoms worn during sleep may be used. The nocturnal emission sample can be drawn up with a syringe from the tip of the condom. Three samples each collected 2 weeks apart are required to obtain representative results. This imposition on the patient is unavoidable because of the substantial sample variation and observer error. To establish whether there is any abnormal sperm – mucus interaction mid-cycle mucus is collected either following intercourse or may be mixed with semen (sperm mucus contact test). If it is impossible to collect mucus at the correct time ethinyl oestradiol (50 μg b.d., 4 days) will induce a similar type of mucus. An abnormal mucus penetration test may draw attention to the need for further assessment of the antibody status. Sperm antibodies are assessed by the immunobead test of sperm (direct) or serum (indirect) (WHO 1992).

Interpretation of semen analysis results

Low volumes suggest incomplete collection, brief abstinence, congenital absence of the vas, ejaculatory duct obstruction or retrograde ejaculation. High volumes over 8 ml, dilute the sperm and create the illusion of low sperm output. It is usually unimportant. Haemospermia is often related to a problem in the prostatic urethra and is rarely important. Slow liquefaction is presumed to reveal defects in accessory organ secretions.

Low sperm concentration ($<20 \times 10^6$ sperm/ml) is referred to as oligospermia (WHO 1992). Controversy exists about this value below which conception becomes difficult: values between 10 and 60×10^6 sperm/ml have been proposed. The average fertile man has 80×10^6/ml (Mallidis et al 1991).

Asthenospermia is defined as sperm motility below 50% or $<25\%$ with rapid linear progressive motility. Spurious results follow exposure to latex, heat, spermicides and delays in delivery or examination of sperm. Most often the result is genuine and accompanies oligospermia, reflecting defective spermatogenesis. Zero (or $<5\%$) motility suggests a sperm tail or mitochondrial defect. Some men who have absent dynein arms in the sperm tail may have generalized cilial defects manifest as sinusitis, bronchiectasis, situs inversus and colour-blindness. These men usually have normal sperm numbers and viability. By contrast, men with necrospermia have $<20\%$ motility and $<30\%$ viability. This may be due to an epididymal disorder in which the storage of sperm is defective (Wilton et al 1988). If these men can ejaculate twice daily for the 4 days prior to ovulation it may be possible to improve motility and viability culminating in conception. Low motility may also result from sperm autoimmunity.

Teratospermia refers to $<30\%$ of sperm showing normal morphology. Percentage of normal sperm morphology is one of the best prognostic factors for IVF. We use the Papanicolau or Shorr stains as these provide satisfactory staining of sperm as well as differentiating leucocytes from sperm precursors. Differential counts of head, mid-piece and tail defects can be made. Additional staining with peroxidase assists the identification of leucocytes. More than 1 million polymorphs/ml is abnormal but there is often a poor correlation with the leucocyte count and culture of organisms. We have found the traditional parameters of genital tract infection such as prostatic tenderness and enlargement, reduced semen volume, lowered pH, reduced prostatic phosphatase and seminal fructose to be unreliable and poorly correlated with positive culture or improvement following empirical antibiotic therapy. We believe this is not a significant problem in most patients.

Hormone assessment

If the FSH is high in azoospermic or severely oligospermic men it suggests a primary defect within the seminiferous epithelium. If the azoospermic man has normal testes and normal FSH he is a candidate for bypass surgery if a remediable obstructive lesion can be defined. Difficulties arise when a man has a low sperm concentration, e.g. 4×10^6/ml, with partial obstruction and seminiferous tubule failure in both testes or partial obstruction of one testis and seminiferous tubule failure of the other. In these testicular biopsy may be necessary.

Men who have small testes with features of incomplete pubertal development or androgen deficiency will need FSH, LH, testosterone and prolactin measured. Those men who have low testosterone without compensatory elevation of LH require hormonal and radiological investigation to exclude a space-occupying lesion in the hypothalamic–pituitary region. If normal they probably have deficient gonadotrophin releasing hormone (GnRH) which is readily treatable. A prolactin assay to detect a pituitary adenoma is essential if the man complains of loss of libido, gynaecomastia or galactorrhoea. Classic symptoms and signs of a pituitary tumour are often absent. Other studies for pituitary lesions, growth hormone (GH), thyroid stimulating hormone (TSH) and thyroxine, cortisol and adrenocorticotrophic hormone (ACTH) may be necessary. Men who present with elevated testosterone may have congenital adrenal hyperplasia in which elevation of serum 17-hydroxyprogesterone is diagnostic. Chromosome analysis may provide the explanation for small testes with marked elevation of FSH and LH. Most of these men have 46XXY (Klinefelter's syndrome) or variants with additional X chromosomes. 46XX men are uncommon but may be normally masculinized. 46XYY men may also have defective spermatogenesis. Cystic fibrosis gene abnormalities may be present in men with congenitally absent vasa (Silber et al 1990, Rojas et al 1992). Respiratory disease may be subtle or absent.

Sperm autoimmunity

In the 7% of men who have sperm antibodies a proportion have genital tract obstruction. In others there may be an associated familial tendency to develop organ-specific auto-antibodies. About 70% of men develop sperm antibodies following vasectomy; these are only important if subsequent vasovasostomy is required. Positive tests do not indicate that the antibodies are invariably responsible for the infertility. If the immunobead binding is <70% IgA to the sperm head, or if there is only binding to the tail tips associated with near-normal mucus penetration, then one should look elsewhere for the cause of infertility. In many instances there is accompanying oligospermia and low motility.

Testis biopsy

As FSH assays provided a biochemical marker for seminiferous tubule failure this technique declined in popularity. In the past decade surgeons have become more adventurous with obstructive lesions, therefore more precise information is required about the adequacy of sperm production than FSH measurements can provide. To avoid general anaesthesia and overnight hospital admission needle aspiration (Menghini) (Mallidis & Baker 1993) or needle core (Tru-cut) biopsies may be taken under local anaesthetic. The key feature of histological assessment is whether spermatogenesis is normal. If so the surgeon is advised to proceed to what may be a meticulous, time-consuming bypass operation or sperm aspiration for IVF.

Ultrasound

Modern ultrasonic instruments can define the scrotal contents better than clinical examination alone, e.g. hydroceles, epididymal cysts and testis tumours (Middleton 1991). Colour Doppler studies help confirm the diagnosis of varicoceles if doubt exists.

Reactive oxygen species

These molecules are generated in excess by defective sperm with increased amounts of cytoplasm and leucocytes, and they may have a deleterious effect on adjacent normal sperm (Wu et al 1989, Iwasaki & Gagnon 1992). Measurement of reactive oxygen species or their effects are currently a research procedure which may become an important routine study.

MANAGEMENT

Gonadotrophin deficiency

FSH and LH may be replaced by exogenous FSH (e.g. Humegon, Organon or Pergonal, Serono) given in a dose of 150 u twice weekly while human chorionic gonadotrophin (hCG) (e.g. equivalent to LH, Pregnyl, CSL Australia or Profasi, Serono) is given at 1500–2000 u twice per week. These doses may be increased for big men or if there is no response. Treatment may be necessary for 18 months in some patients. Progress is monitored by evidence of androgen secretion, testicular volume and semen analyses. At the outset the patient should be warned that it is usually a protracted exercise. As the deficiency of FSH may be minor hCG alone for up to 6 months may overcome the infertility. Hypothalamic disorders resulting in GnRH deficiency may be treated by means of exogenous, pulsatile GnRH delivered subcutaneously from a battery-operated pump worn in a vest pocket. The one agent in small doses (up to 500 μg per day) stimulates both FSH and LH. It is economical, safe, but cumbersome. About half of these men produce children. Gonadotrophin suppression occurs in athletes who use illicit androgens and anabolic agents. Usually, once they desist the sperm concentration rises over about 6 months.

Sperm autoimmunity

Treatment with prednisolone either continuously, at 50 mg per day for 3–6 months, or intermittently at 25–75 mg per day for 10 days each month, has been shown to improve fertility in controlled trials, but only 25–40% achieve a pregnancy (Hendry et al 1990). Pregnancy may also occur with IVF after short-term glucocorticoid therapy or with cryopreserved semen collected during glucocorticoid treatment. The man must be informed of the serious side-effects such as avascular necrosis of the head of the femur. Management of these couples may be complicated by the wife's compromised fertility.

Coital disorders

Infertility may disturb the man's perception of his masculinity, making him prone to performance anxiety. This may be compounded by anxiety about basal body temperature charts, an anxious wife or the need to provide semen specimens on demand for analysis or assisted reproductive technology. Gonadotrophin therapy for those with hypogonadism may dramatically improve the situation. As testosterone concentrations rise towards the normal range in these men, potency improves but may be complicated by the emotional difficulties of a postponed adolescence.

Ambivalence about having children may be manifest as psychogenic impotence. Diabetes, spinal cord injury or disease, or trauma to pelvic nerves, may declare themselves through ejaculatory or erectile dysfunction. Some healthy young men have erectile failure for no apparent reason. Prostaglandin E_1 administered by injection into the corpora cavernosa of the penis of all of these men is an effective way of achieving an erection. For the reluctant lover a pharmacologically induced erection, which is obvious to his wife, may compound his embarrassment and complicate the relationship. A simpler approach is to show the couple how to transfer an ejaculate collected by masturbation into the vagina by means of a long 1 ml syringe.

Ejaculatory failure may be circumvented by collecting nocturnal emissions in a non-toxic (silastic) condom and transferring it on awakening to the vagina. If the sperm is passing retrogradely into the bladder, especially in diabetic men, medications to tighten the sphincter (brompheniramine, an antihistamine or ephedrine — an α-adrenergic receptor agonist) may help. Intercouse with a full bladder achieves the same objective in some men. Strong mechanical vibration applied to the inferior aspect of the tip of the penis, beneath the glans, may trigger ejaculation (Wheeler et al 1988). If this fails an electro-ejaculation probe inserted into the rectum to stimulate efferent nerve fibres passing from the spinal cord to the genitalia may be successful (Randolf et al 1990). A light general anaesthetic is required and the ejaculate is not invariably good following the first session of stimulation. Concentration and motility improve in some men on subsequent occasions. Some of these men have retrograde ejaculation which may be overcome by alkalinizing the urine (sodium bicarbonate 3.5 g four times per day for 3 days) and retrieval by catheter.

The urine is centrifuged immediately and the precipitated sperm are transferred to a tissue culture medium for insemination. Such sperm are invariably poor in terms of motility, concentration and fertilizing capacity. It is imperative that the chances of conception are enhanced by accurate timing of insemination at ovulation using mucus assessment, urinary LH measurement (Clearplan, Fisons) or plasma LH, progesterone and E_2 concentrations.

Genital tract inflammation

Bilateral mumps orchitis in adulthood is almost invariably followed by permanent infertility. Untreated or resistant gonococcal epididymitis may result in obstructive azoospermia. More often the presumed genital tract infection is much more subtle. It is usually asymptomatic, evident only by an excess of leucocytes in the semen.

Varicoceles

The clinical relevance of this disorder remains controversial. Varicoceles occur in 25% of men assessed for infertility and in a similar proportion of fertile men. They appear after puberty, and hypogonadal men are less likely to have a varicocele. Men with large testes or tall men are more likely to have a varicocele. Almost all are left-sided and the accompanying testis is smaller and softer than its counterpart (Baker et al 1985, Chehval & Purcell 1992).

There is no assurance that varicocele ligation will improve fertility and the patient should be aware of the limited prospects of success. Discomfort due to the varicocele or a solitary testis surrounded by a varicocele makes the decision to have a ligation easier. General anaesthesia and protracted wound healing can be avoided by X-ray-controlled venous catheter occlusion devices.

Combined sclerosant infusion and insertion of a thrombogenic coil in scrotal varicosities may achieve comparable venous occlusion to surgical ligation. A favourable response should not be anticipated before 3 months. In the event of improved semen quality, samples should be stored frozen during the non-fertile phase of the ovulatory cycle in the event that the better sperm quality is not sustained. Continuing improvement has been reported for up to 12 months. We remain pessimistic about this treatment modality, especially if the sperm concentration is very low and the FSH is high.

General management

This deals with men who have normal semen, idiopathic oligospermia, or poor morphology or motility for which no specific treatment is available. It is important to review the wife's fertility, coital timing, technique and psychological aspects of the relationship. Those women presenting later in life after their careers have been established or after prolonged infertility are less likely to conceive. Adverse psychological reactions to poor prognoses are common. Empathy, information, education and time allow them to cope and make rational decisions about their management. We stress the need for them to seek solace from one another rather than reject the partner who appears to be responsible. Irrespective of the severity of the oligospermia they ought to have intercourse during the ovulatory phase, i.e. the 'conception window' on days 13, 14 and 15. Many men with sperm concentrations below 5×10^6/ml father children. It is therefore imperative that the relationship does not falter on the false premise that less than 20×10^6 sperm/ml indicates that he is solely responsible for the infertility. While those men who have chromosomal defects have only a remote possibility of impregnating their wives, we counsel them to continue trying while considering other options such as donor insemination.

If the woman recognizes mittleschmertz (pain of ovulation), the increased cervical mucus volume and tackiness, accurate timing with the aid of a basal body temperature chart is not difficult. The urinary LH detection kits (e.g. Clearplan) are simple to use and have been a very useful educational device for women endeavouring to time ovulation for coitus or other treatment. It has been particularly useful for country folk who cannot attend the clinic.

Empirical treatment

The following treatments have had enthusiastic advocates: androgen 're-bound' therapy, weak androgens to stimulate accessory gland function without gonadotrophin suppression, hCG with or without FSH, anti-oestrogens such as clomiphene, amino acids, vitamins, zinc, herbs, cold baths and testicular coolers. They have either not been subjected to scientific scrutiny, or if they have, failed to survive. It is sobering to note that men who received human pituitary FSH and hCG on an empirical basis two decades ago are currently being warned that they may develop Creutzfeldt–Jakob disease. Placing 'washed husband's sperm' high in the uterine cavity (AIH) has had mixed reports, with controlled trials failing to support its use.

In vitro fertilization

Assisted reproductive technology including IVF has assumed a more important role for the infertile male. If $>2 \times 10^6$ motile sperm can be harvested from an ejaculate the success rate is acceptable, around 15%. GIFT and modifications of this procedure have been reported to give variable results; definition of their role is awaited. A test sample of sperm should be evaluated prior to treatment in the event that treatable infection is evident or the husband cannot produce a sample on demand. It may be prudent to freeze-store sperm in the event that the sample provided on the day of fertilization is unsuitable. Persistent zero motility or specific structural defects are indicative of a poor outcome. If IVF is not feasible, donor insemination should be considered.

The above methods have provided the means to assess various sperm parameters and procedures alleged to improve sperm function. IVF fertilization rates improve from 20% to 60% as the percentage of morphologically normal sperm increases from <5% to >50%. With respect to motility, average straight-line velocity and average linearity of motion were the most significant predictors of IVF success. The proportion of sperm with intact acrosomes in semen is also a positive predictor. Various zona pellucida binding studies have been developed using oocytes which failed to fertilize. It can be estimated whether a comparable number of the patient's sperm bind to the zona compared with normal donor sperm. While these tests are powerful determinants of IVF success they are not generally available. If normal semen is used, up to 60% of oocytes fertilize and cleave in the context of IVF. Should the semen contain <20% of sperm with normal morphology only 35% of oocytes fertilize and cleave normally. Success is lower if there is the added problem of low motile sperm concentration. Once fertilization occurs with abnormal semen the outcome for the pre-embryo appears to be similar to that of pre-embryos obtained with normal semen. This is both in terms of normal babies born and pregnancy wastage. Complete failure of fertilization is almost always caused by male factors. It warrants careful review of the morphology and gamete interaction.

Micromanipulation

Failure of conventional IVF has led to attempts to broach the barrier of the zona pellucida by placing the sperm under the zona (subzonal insemination (SUZI), Kola et al 1990) or by rupturing the zona (partial zona dissection (PZD), Cohen et al 1988, Fishel et al 1992, Jean et al 1992) and allowing the sperm to enter. Success has been infrequent but fertilization (20%) and pregnancy rates (5%) are improving. With these techniques polyspermy is common (10%). Intracytoplasmic injection (ICSI) has been reported to produce higher fertilization rates (50%) even with severe sperm abnormalities, zero motility and total teratospermia.

Donor sperm

Up to 1 in 200 babies born in those countries using donor gametes are from artificial insemination or IVF with frozen donor sperm. Indications include sterility or chronic subfertility in the male (Kovacs et al 1988). Many couples cannot accept the notion of donor sperm until IVF with the husband's sperm and other treatments have failed. Donor sperm may also be used with IVF as a back-up if the husband's sperm fails to fertilize oocytes in routine IVF. Fresh donor sperm is not recommended because of the need to quarantine sperm for 6 months after collection to allow time for antibodies to develop to the HIV virus. This interval would also permit symptoms and signs of sexually transmitted disease to become apparent. Donors are checked by history and examination for any trait or disease which may be transmitted to the child. Young men (20–45 years) with excellent sperm which will freeze well are chosen. Urethral swabs and blood are collected for screening tests and the physical features are documented. 'Known donors' refers to friends or relatives the couple choose to provide sperm. Parties to such arrangements require very careful counselling and legal advice. Also identical screening procedures for anonymous donors are used. Insemination is timed to ovulation as described above. It may be performed by the consultant, a specially trained nurse, family doctor or, in some instances, the husband. Success relates to the recipient's fertility, usually 10–15% per month for the first 6 months, so that about 50% of women are pregnant by 6 months. For women who repeatedly fail to conceive there is a trend to administer ovulation induction agents or resort to IVF. Such women can be assured of an 80% chance of having a child within 2 years.

Counselling

Skilled counselling is now generally available and in some centres is obligatory for assisted reproductive procedures. Clinicians tend to deal with this aspect of management superficially and the couple are given the opportunity of asking questions about the procedure from someone who may be less intimidating. They need guidance about discussing the paternity of their child. Reassurance should be given about the insignificant risk of consanguineous marriage of their child with another individual from the same donor.

Prevention of male infertility

Avoidance of physicochemical noxious agents (e.g. ionizing radiation, lead and benzene) are made possible by community health and education measures. Prompt treatment of gonorrhoea may prevent epididymal obstruction. Undescended testes which are not brought down do not have normal spermatogenesis. Men whose testes are medically or surgically brought into the scrotum do not necessarily become fertile. More research is required to resolve how and when this disorder is best treated (Puri & O'Donnell 1988). Mumps virus vaccines are now available. Prophylactic ligation of varicoceles in young men (Laven et al 1992) is as controversial as it is in those with established infertility. At least in this group it may be prudent to store frozen sperm. Another area in which cryopreservation is underutilized is prior to vasectomy. Our experience of storing sperm prior to orchidectomy or chemotherapy for malignant disease has been disappointing. The samples are poor and post-thaw motility is low. Other possibilities for sperm storage include drug therapy of nephritis, prostatic disease, psoriasis and inflammatory bowel disease. Sperm stored in the acute phase of mumps orchitis will be contamined with the virus and could only be given to an immune woman. Rarely, men with Young's syndrome have fathered children before the obstruction develops; thus young men with bronchiectasis should be offered sperm cryopreservation.

CONCLUSION

Male infertility has been neglected until the past few decades. Now that female infertility has been defined, and in many instances treated successfully, it is timely to focus on the male. While most causes of male infertility are incurable there have been major advances in basic knowledge and research which will foster development of better diagnostic and therapeutic measures.

KEY POINTS FOR CLINICAL PRACTICE

1. Assess the couple rather than individual partners
2. No sperm, small testes, high FSH — poor prognosis
3. No sperm, small testes, low FSH — try gonadotrophin treatment
4. No sperm, normal testes, normal FSH — bypass surgery
5. Sperm antibodies positive with no mucus penetration — glucocorticoids
6. Spontaneous pregnancy rate is significant especially with young women, brief duration of infertility and better semen
7. If all of the above fail resort to IVF or donor sperm.

REFERENCES

Baker H W G, Burger H G, de Krester D M et al 1985 Testicular vein ligation and fertility in men with varicoceles. Br Med J 291: 1678–1680
Baker H W G, Burger H G, de Kretser D M et al 1986 Relative incidence of etiological disorders in male infertility. In: Santen R J, Swerdloff R S (eds) Male reproductive dysfunction: diagnosis and management of hypogonadism, infertility and impotence. Dekker, New York, pp 341–372
Chehval M J, Purcell M H 1992 Deterioration of semen parameters over time in men with untreated varicocele: evidence of progressive testicular damage. Fertil Steril 57: 174–177
Cohen J, Malter H, Fehilly C et al 1988 Implantation of embryos after partial opening of oocyte zona pellucida to facilitate sperm penetration. Lancet ii: 162
Comhaire F H, de Krester D M, Farley T M et al 1987 Towards more objectivity in diagnosis and management of male infertility. Int J Androl (Suppl) 7: 1–53
Fishel S, Timson J, Lisi F et al 1992 Evaluation of 225 patients undergoing subzonal insemination for the procurement of fertilization in vitro. Fertil Steril 58: 840–849
Greenhall E, Vessey M 1990 The prevalence of subfertility: a review of the current confusion and a report of two new studies. Fertil Steril 54: 978–983
Henderson, J, Baker H W G, Hanna P J 1986 Occupationally related male infertility: a review. Clin Reprod Fertil 4: 87–106
Hendry W F, Hughes L, Scamell G et al 1990 Comparison of prednisolone and placebo in subfertile men with antibodies to spermatozoa. Lancet 335: 85–88
Iwasaki A, Gagnon C 1992 Formation of reactive oxygen species in spermatozoa of infertile patients. Fertil Steril 57: 409–416
Jean M, L'Hermite A, Barriere P et al 1992 Utility of zona pellucida drilling in cases of

severe semen alterations in man. Fertil Steril 57: 591–596

Kola I, Lachman O, Jansen R P S et al 1990 Chromosomal analysis of human oocytes fertilized by microinjection of spermatozoa into the perivitelline space. Hum Reprod 5: 575–577

Kovacs G, Baker G, Burger H G et al 1988 AID with cryopreserved semen: a decade of experience. Br J Obstet Gynaecol 95: 354–360

Laven J Ŝ E, te Velde E T, Haans L C F et al 1992 Effects of varicocele treatment in adolescents: a randomized study. Fertil Steril 58: 756–762

Mallidis C, Baker H W G Fine needle tissue aspiration biopsy (FNTAB) of the testis. Fertil Steril (in press)

Mallidis C, Howard E J, Baker H W G 1991 Variation of semen quality in normal men. Int J Androl 14: 99–107

Middleton W D 1991 Scrotal sonography in 1991. Ultrasound Q 9: 61–87

Oldereid N B, Rui H, Clausen O P et al 1989 Cigarette smoking and human sperm quality assessed by laser–Doppler spectroscopy and DNA flow cyometry. J Reprod Fertil 86: 731–736

Puri P, O'Donnell B 1988 Semen analysis of patients who had orchidopexy at or after seven years of age. Lancet ii: 1051–1052

Randolf J F Jr, Ohl D A, Bennett C J et al 1990 Combined electroejaculation and in vitro fertilization in the evaluation and treatment of anejaculatory infertility. J In Vitro Fert Embryo Transf 7: 58–62

Rojas F J, La A-T, Ord J et al 1992 Penetration of zona free hamster oocytes using human sperm aspirated from the epididymis of men with congenital absence of the vas deferens: comparison with human in vitro fertilization. Fertil Steril 58: 1000–1005

Silber S J, Ord T, Balmaceda J et al 1990 Congenital absence of the vas deferens: the fertilizing capacity of human epididymal sperm. N Engl J Med 323: 1788–1792

Wheeler J S Jr, Walter J S, Culkin D J et al 1988 Idiopathic anejaculation treated by vibratory stimulation. Fertil Steril 50: 377–379

WHO laboratory manual for the examination of human semen and sperm–cervical mucus interaction 1992 3rd edition. Cambridge University Press

Wilton L J, Temple-Smith P D, Baker H W G et al 1988 Human male infertility caused by degeneration and death of sperm in the epididymis. Fertil Steril 49: 1052–1058

Wu F C, Aitken R J, Ferguson A 1989 Inflammatory bowel disease and male infertility: effects of sulfasalazine and 5-aminosalicylic acid on sperm-fertilizing capacity and reactive oxygen species generation. Fertil Steril 52: 842–845

7

Recurrent abortion: a review

C. Barry-Kinsella   R. F. Harrison

Recurrent abortion, defined as three consecutive pregnancies ending sponta-neously before the 20th week of gestation, is an uncommon condition, with an estimated risk of some 0.4% and an observed risk of 0.8% (Huisjes 1990). From a clinical point of view, couples are often extremely distressed and look for both an adequate explanation and preventive treatment in the next pregnancy. Large gaps remain in our knowledge of early prenatal develop-ment. Further scientific studies are required to elucidate possible causes of single and recurrent abortion.

Of the many causes of recurrent abortion that have been cited, few have specific effective therapy (Glass & Goldbus 1978). In the majority of cases, no apparent fetal or parental abnormality is found. Empirical therapies have been advocated, but some have been subsequently shown to be harmful (Herbst et al 1971). Few therapies have been evaluated in well-designed placebo-controlled trials and often benefit is suggested where none may exist.

Questions have been asked about the formidable lists of causes that have evolved (DeCherney & Polan 1984) and studies are now taking into account the known overall spontaneous cure rates of over 50%.

CAUSES OF RECURRENT ABORTION

The cause of individual abortions for a couple with recurrent pregnancy loss is not always the same (Huisjes 1990). More than one factor may exist and thorough investigation (Chamberlain 1982) often fails to reveal a common theme. Nevertheless, for the purposes of this review, each cause will be examined as if it had the potential to be the sole aetiological factor. No distinction has been made between women with a primary or secondary habitual abortion history even though the prognosis in the latter is likely to be more favourable (DeCherney & Polan 1984).

Potential causes of habitual abortion have been classified in many different ways. This review divides them into two groups: *doubtful*, where current data suggest a loose association (Chamberlain 1982) and *possible*, where the association has more scientific validity but the final proof is lacking.

Doubtful

Anatomical abnormalities of the uterus

Retroversion. Traditional thinking suggests that backward tilt of the uterus may cause a miscarriage. Although a gravid fixed retroverted uterus may become incarcerated within the pelvis during the first trimester, no evidence suggests that this process or retroversion itself jeopardizes a pregnancy. The significance of a retroverted uterus as an aetiological factor in pregnancy loss must be questioned in modern obstetric practice.

Intrauterine adhesions. This condition, first described by Asherman (1948), may be suspected by a history of light or absent menstruation and confirmed by intrauterine filling defects visualized at hysterogram or synechae demonstrated at hysteroscopy. Intrauterine adhesions are more likely to cause infertility than habitual abortion. Various treatment options are available (Jansen 1982). In an uncontrolled study (Jewlewicz et al 1976), in which many of the 36 women had had recurrent abortions, 50% conception rate and 16% uncomplicated full-term delivery rate was reported after treatment.

Infection

A number of organisms have been implicated as causing habitual abortion. These include toxoplasmosis, listeria, brucella, chlamydia, mycoplasmas, herpes simplex and cytomegalovirus (Chamberlain 1982, Stirrat 1983, Charles & Larsen 1990). Many of these organisms are, however, found commonly in the vagina. Toxoplasmosis could possibly cause abortion by invading the placenta or by transplacentally affecting the fetus, but this usually occurs later in the pregnancy and does not appear to be a significant factor for the habitual aborter. Southern (1982) found a positive dye test for toxoplasmosis in 20% of habitual aborters and in 21.3% of controls. *Listeria monocytogenes* has been shown to be associated with habitual abortion in animals but not in the human. In some studies (Caspe et al 1972) evidence is presented that mycoplasmas are a causative factor but other studies (Harrison et al 1979) have found to the contrary.

An infective agent per se or the resultant high fever (as in the case of malaria) can cause a woman to abort, but no definitive evidence has shown that any specific agent causes habitual abortion. Even syphilis (Harter & Benirsche 1976), which is capable of penetrating the placental barrier in early pregnancy, and which is still associated with sporadic spontaneous abortion, after treatment has been eliminated as a cause of habitual abortion.

Further work, from well-designed prospective studies of culture results, could recategorize infective organisms from the doubtful to the possibly significant group (Charles & Larsen 1990, Southern 1982) .

Endocrine/metabolic disease

Although rare, the patient with an untreated adrenal hyperplasia may have an increased chance of recurrent abortion (Chamberlain 1982). The role of hypothyroidism (Jones & Deys 1951) in recurrent abortion is now challenged and definitive proof is considered lacking. Nevertheless, it is good clinical practice to look for signs of hypothyroidism and to treat this when found.

Carbohydrate intolerance and diabetes mellitus have long been thought to cause habitual abortion. In women with poorly controlled diabetes there is a higher risk of congenital abnormality, and polycystic ovary syndrome (PCOS) patients with hyperinsulinaemia have abortion rates higher than other infertile women. The available evidence suggests that diabetes mellitus is not a cause of recurrent abortion (Huisjes 1990). Thus glucose tolerance testing in such women has become redundant, except where there is a high index of clinical suspicion from the history or physical examination.

In maternal diseases (Huisjes 1990) such as congenital hypofibrinogenaemia, factor XIII deficiency, phenylketonuria and glucose-6-phosphate dehydrogenase deficiency, evidence suggests an increased risk. These abnormalities are rarely encountered and convincing evidence is difficult to obtain.

The doubtful category must also include the more commonly found diseases such as chronic intestinal problems, Crohn's disease, sickle cell disease, psychiatric disturbance and endometriosis. The evidence supporting endometriosis as a cause is based on an increased abortion rate found in a selected population of women who later developed endometriosis (Pittaway & Karlsten Wentz 1984). The increased levels of $PGF_{2\alpha}$ found in women with endometriosis are the suggested mechanism. However, the risk of abortion appears inversely related to the severity of the disease (Wheler et al 1983).

Exogenous causes

Certain environmental factors have been suspected as increasing the risk of spontaneous abortion (Hemminki et al 1990). Exposure to herbicide spraying, living near electromagnetic fields and sources of radiation have been more noted for the amount of media attention generated than warranted by the available scientific evidence.

While drug use and abuse may cause problems in an index pregnancy, there is no evidence that long-term implications are carried through to other pregnancies. Alcohol, smoking and street drugs (Stirrat 1983) have linked with habitual abortion but a multifactorial situation (Harrison 1986) usually exists.

Occupational hazards (Hemminki et al 1990) such as the frequent inhalation of anaesthetic gases, exposure to solvents, heavy metals and industrial chemicals have all shown an association with habitual loss in some studies but not in others. Early data suggested these positive associations, but later, better-designed studies produced negative results. This was shown with anaesthetic gases (Hemminki et al 1986). The Royal College of Obstetricians and Gynaecologists has stated that visual display units do not appear to effect pregnancy outcome.

Possible

General disease

Wilson's disease is a rare disorder of copper metabolism (Huisjes 1990) which is diagnosed when the serum caeruloplasmin level is below 20 mmol/l or when an increase in copper excretion is found in the urine after administration of penicillamine. Such women will abort (Scheinberg & Sternlieb 1975) if not treated with this drug.

Systemic lupus erythematosus (SLE) may also be a possible reason for habitual abortion (Huisjes 1990). This does not, however, appear to be true in all cases and may depend on the activity and severity of the disease (Imbasciati et al 1984). This is possibly because of complement consumption in the placenta (Trennan et al 1978) or cross-reaction of lymphocytotoxic antibodies with the trophoblast (Bresnihan et al 1977). Timing of pregnancies during remission and active treatment of flare activity may pay dividends and when a pregnancy occurs it should be treated as high risk.

The presence of the lupus anticoagulant even in the absence of clinical SLE also appears to be associated with habitual abortion. Where anticardiolipin antibodies exist, which are closely related to those responsible for lupus anticoagulant activity, the same situation appears to prevail. This subject is dealt with in Chapter 2.

Fetal abnormalities of genetic origin

The majority of early spontaneous abortions are chromosomally abnormal and most occur as a non-recurrent chance phenomenon (Lauritsen 1976). The most common abnormalities are the autosomal trisomies, followed by monosomy X and polyploidy (DeCherney & Polan 1984). However, there appears to be an increased risk of chromosomal abnormality in a subsequent pregnancy if the first abortion was chromosomally abnormal (Boue & Boue 1973). Many genetic disorders have multifactorial influences (Davison & Burn 1973). It is also theoretically possible that non-chromosome causes such as decreased DNA content of the spermatozoal head (Chamberlain 1982) may exert influence in this way.

It is important to evaluate the chromosomal complement of both partners for an abnormality. An abnormal karyotype will be diagnosed in one or other partner in 5–7% of these couples. Banding techniques are necessary to identify translocations. The incidence of such aberrations in couples presenting with habitual abortion is around 3%. This is several times the expected norm. Commonly these are reciprocal translocations (two-thirds) with one-third being a Robertsonian translocation (Tho et al 1979). The carrier is usually the female partner but both karyotypes must be examined.

Where a defect is identified, at present no effective therapy exists other than considering relevant gamete donation to circumvent the problem. The couple should receive experienced genetic counselling to inform them of the possibility of successful outcome the next time. Such an approach may also help to alleviate the stress that habitual abortion couples experience.

Uterine anatomical defect

Body. Abnormal growth or fusion in utero of the Mullerian system can give rise to a variety of uterine mis-shapes (Jones 1957). The overall incidence has been calculated at between 0.1% (Glass & Goldbus 1978) and 3.5% (DeCherney & Polan 1984). The intrauterine exposure to diethylstilboestrol (DES) may have increased this anomaly. These figures are likely to be an underestimation; for many women the uterine shape will not cause any problem and will not be diagnosed (Jones 1957).

The type of uterine abnormality has been correlated to incidence of habitual abortion (Craig 1973). The worst prognosis is apparently in women with a single uterine horn or a bicornuate uterus. While this may simply reflect the fact that such abnormalities are seemingly more common, they are also the most likely to provide the implanting embryo with a poor blood supply, given that a septum is usually composed of more fibrous tissue than uterine muscle.

Surgery, approached either transabdominally or via the hysteroscope, which aims to restore the uterine cavity to 'normality' is reported to provide excellent results (Craig 1972). Such operations are, however, not without complications.

Fibromyomata. The true incidence of fibroids is unknown. They are common tumours in older women and those from Negro races. A deficiency of the endometrium may certainly arise near the site of a submucous fibroid, and this could cause early miscarriage if implantation occurs in the affected area where the blood supply is abnormal (DeCherney & Polan 1984). If another cause for recurrent miscarriage is not found, myomectomy may be advisable. Myomectomy or hysteroscopic resection has the potential complications such as adhesion formation which could decrease the chances of further conception.

Cervix. The circular muscle fibres at and around the internal cervical os may be congenitally weak, damaged iatrogenically or traumatized by labour. Although cervical incompetence is a recognized cause of habitual abortion, controversy remains about the incidence, diagnosis and treatment. The condition is often over-diagnosed. A suspicion of cervical weakness relies mainly on history and diagnosis on hysterosalpingography or the easy passage of large dilators through the cervix. However, a definitive diagnosis may have to wait until pregnancy occurs. Ultrasound findings of dilatation or shortening of the cervix are suggestive but digital palpation of the cervix for premature dilatation and effacement is necessary for diagnosis.

This wait-and-see approach in doubtful cases may prevent unnecessary intervention which involves some form of cervical cerclage. Where a patient has a clear-cut history of severe trauma to the cervix and/or a number of mid-trimester abortions in which no other cause has been found, cervical cerclage should be performed. The optimum time for this is around the 12th to 14th week when fetal viability has been demonstrated; occasionally the history may demand earlier intervention. The surgery aims to position the suture accurately to correct the weakened cervical internal os. Many varieties of operation have been used both per abdomen and per vaginum; good results may be obtained using mersilene tape (Murphy et al 1978) and a modified Shirodkar technique (Shirodar 1955).

Immunological

How the fetus is accepted immunologically by the mother remains unknown (Kurt 1980, Houwert de Jong et al 1990). Acceptance may reflect either a failure of immunological response by the maternal immune system or alternatively active immunosuppression. The absence of the major histocompatible HLA antigens has been noted on the syncytiotrophoblast, but class 1 HLA ABC and class II HLA DR antigens have been found (Sunderland et al 1981). It has been proposed that maternal recognition of trophoblast–lymphocyte cross-reactive (TLX) antigens and production of antibodies to TLX — the so-called 'blocking' antigen — is responsible for fetal survival.

Couples with habitual abortion are more likely than expected to share HLA antigens, thus preventing trophoblast recognition and the failure to generate the appropriate beneficial 'blocking' antibodies (Beer 1986). Based on this theory many centres have immunized women with trophoblast, paternal and unrelated lymphocytes to induce this putative response (Taylor & Falk 1981). Data from the first randomized prospective controlled study using partner's lymphocytes was encouraging (Mowbray et al 1985) but has not been confirmed. Questions have been posed about the scientific validity (Adinolfi 1986) of this approach and there is concern about cross-infection and long-term immunosuppression. While this treatment has been widely used, 'immunotherapy' requires further investigation by well-designed multicentred controlled trials.

Hormonal

Traditionally the diagnosis of endocrine dysfunction has been cited where either no other cause for recurrent abortion has been found, where the corpus luteum deficiency is suspected or where progesterone levels have been shown to be low. This diagnosis has been made despite the fact, in the latter case in particular, that the hormone abnormality may be the effect rather than the cause of imminent pregnancy loss. Oestrogens and progesterone are important for the maintenance of early pregnancy (Csapa & Pulkkinen 1978). Consequently their deficiency has been considered as a cause for habitual abortion. Such a deficiency is difficult to prove, and to all intents and purposes cannot be diagnosed. Nevertheless, hormone supplementation has been used to prevent recurrent pregnancy loss, but oestrogen supplements have unacceptable side-effects (Herbst et al 1971), and gestogens and progesterone are no better than placebo (Shearman & Garrett 1963, Reinjnders et al 1988).

Human chorionic gonadotrophin (hCG) in vivo stimulates both the corpus luteum (Savard et al 1964) and early fetoplacental endocrine function (Varangot et al 1965). It has been shown to prolong the life of the corpus luteum (Brown & Bradbury 1947), enabling it to continue to secrete oestrogen/progesterone until this is taken over by the placenta. A placentotrophic effect has been demonstrated in vitro (Diczfalusy & Troen 1961), with increased steroid production, and steroidogenesis has been stimulated (LeMaire et al 1968). In the light of this information exogenous hCG administration has been used to prevent early pregnancy demise.

The dosage regimen for hCG is uncertain (Dukelow 1979); a poor correlation exists between plasma hCG levels and steroid secretions of oestrogen and progesterone (Yoshimi et al 1969). The circulating endogenous hCG level is 50 000 mIU/l, and an injection of 5000 IU/ml will increase this by 2500 mIU/ml (Eshkol 1985).

Various dose regimens in uncontrolled studies have shown positive results. The first placebo-controlled study (Harrison 1985) demonstrated that hCG was significantly better than placebo. The numbers studied were, however, small and in the subsequent larger multicentric trial (Harrison et al 1993) no statistical significance was demonstrated between hCG and placebo. A previous metanalysis of the available data (Prendiville 1991) has shown hCG to be better than placebo.

INVESTIGATION OF RECURRENT ABORTION

Ideally the couple should be involved in all stages of investigations. History, physical examination and a limited number of relevant investigations are likely to reveal very quickly whether any possible aetiological factor is present.

The past reproductive history, noting the gestation at which a pregnancy loss occurred, is particularly relevant as many abortions associated with chromosomal abnormalities occur early, whereas those associated with cervical or uterine abnormality usually present late. In this latter regard, confirmatory hysterography or hysteroscopy may be helpful.

The past medical history may indicate relevant diseases, and an evaluation of the lifestyle, environment and specific drug therapies may reveal possibilities that need further exploration. A menstrual history and physical examination may provide clues to endocrine abnormalities and suggest specific hormone investigations. These are particularly relevant for women with polycystic ovarian disease where high baseline LH levels have been associated with early pregnancy loss.

Serological tests for SLE, anticardiolipin antibodies and lupus anticoagulant, even in the absence of clinical disease, should be performed. In both partners, a chromosomal analysis including G banding is advisable. Testing for specific infections is not cost-effective and as yet there is no specific investigation which will diagnose a hormonal or an immunological factor in clinical practice. Thus in the majority of cases firm diagnoses cannot be made.

Unfortunately, occasionally an equivocal result is obtained from these investigations, underlying the uncertainty that exists about this condition. It is important that the couple understand that this result may not necessarily explain their pregnancy loss.

TREATMENT

When a specific abnormality is found, such as a relevant chromosome aberration in one partner, it may not be possible to suggest specific therapy other than counselling. In some situations such as cervical incompetence or uterine abnormalities where surgical treatment is available, the benefits need to be weighed against possible side-effects. However, when no cause has been found the clinician finds himself in a dilemma. He has the option of providing tender loving care and reassuring ultrasound scans during the next pregnancy or alternatively of providing empirical treatment. When the informed couple choose the latter course of action, there are two options: immunotherapy or hCG supplementation (Stray Pedersen & Stray Pedersen 1984). As with other forms of treatment offered to the habitually aborting couple, they must be aware that the placebo effect is extremely high and the potential benefits must be weighed against the potential risks.

CONCLUSIONS

Providing reassurance and tender loving care may suffice for couples who abort for the first or second time. However, with recurrent abortion this approach is less likely to be acceptable. Full investigation is indicated but in the majority of cases no explanation will be found. Until more knowledge is available from large controlled trials the couple should be discouraged from empirical treatment (Regan 1991).

REFERENCES

Adinolfi M 1986 Recurrent abortion. Follicular abortion: sharing and the deliberate immunisation with partner cells. A controversial topic. Hum Reprod 1: 45–48
Asherman J G 1948 Amenorrhoea traumatica (atretica). J Obstet Gynaecol Br Empire 55: 23–30
Beer A E 1986 New horizons in the diagnosis evaluation and therapy of recurrent spontaneous abortion. Clin Obstet Gynaecol 13: 115–124
Boue J, Boue A 1973 Hum Genitik 19: 275
Bresnihan B N, Oliver R R, Gregor R M et al 1977 Immunological mechanisms for spontaneous abortion in system lupus erythomatosis. Lancet ii: 1205–1207
Brown W E, Bradbury J M 1947 A study of the physiologic action of human chorionic

hormone: the production of pseudopregnancy in women by chorionic hormone. Am J Obstet Gynecol 53: 749–757

Caspe E, Solmon F, Sompolinsky D 1972 Isr J Med Sci 8: 123

Chamberlain G 1982 Recurrent miscarriage and pre-term labour. In: Harley TMG (ed) Clinics in obstetrics and gynaecology, Vol. 9. Saunders, London, pp 115–130.

Charles D, Larsen B 1990 Spontaneous abortion as a result of infection. In: Huisjes M J, Lind T (eds) Clinics in obstetrics and gynaecology: early pregnancy failure. Churchill Livingstone, Edinburgn, pp 161–176

Craig C 1973 Congenital abnormality of the uterus and fetal wastage. S Afr Med J 122: 2000–2005

Csapa A I, Pulkkinen M 1978 Indispensability of the human corpus luteum in the maintenance of early pregnancy: leutoectomy evidence. Obstet Gynaecol Survey 33: 69–81

Davison E V, Burn J 1973 Genetic causes of early pregnancy loss. Hum Genitik 19: 55–78

DeCherney A, Polan M L 1984 Evaluation and management of habitual abortion. Br J Hosp Med April: 261–268

Diczfalusy E, Troen T 1961 Endocrine functions of human placenta. Vitam Horm 19: 229–311

Dukelow R 1979 Human chorionic gonadotrophin induction of ovulation in the squirrel monkey. Science 206: 234–235

Eshkol I 1985 Personal communication

Glass R H, Goldbus M S 1978 Habitual abortion. Fertil Steril 29: 257–265

Harrison R F 1985 Treatment of habitual abortion with human chorionic gonadotropin: results of open and placebo-controlled studies. Eur J Obstet Gynaecol Reprod Biol 20: 159–168

Harrison R F 1986 The use of non-essential drugs, alcohol and cigarettes during pregnancy. Irish Med J 79: 338–441

Harrison R F, Hurley R, de Louvois J 1979 Genital mycoplasmas and birth weight in offspring of primigravid women. Am J Obstet Gynecol 133: 201–203

Harrison et al 1993 Human chorionic gonadotrophin HCG in the management of recurrent abortion: results of a multicentre placebo controlled study. Eur J Obstet Gynaecol Reprod Biol (in press)

Harter C A, Benirsche E K 1976 Fetal syphilis in the first trimester. Am J Obstet Gynecol 124: 705–711

Hemminki K, Lindbolm M L, Taskien H 1986 Transplacental toxicity of environmental chemicals, enviuronmental causes and correlates of spontaneous abortion, malformations and childhood cancer. In: Milunsky A, Friedman E A, Gluck L (eds) Advances in perinatal medicine, Vol 5. Plenum Press, New York, pp 43–91

Hemminki K, Hemminki E, Lindbohm M L, Taskien H 1990 Exogenous causes of spontaneous abortion. In: Huisjes H J, Lind T (eds) Clinics in obstetrics and gynaecology: early pregnancy failure. Churchill Livingstone, Edinburgh, pp 177–195

Herbst A L, Ulfelder H, Poskanzer D G 1971 Adenocarcinoma of the vagina: association of maternal stilboestrol therapy with tumour appearances in young women. N Engl J Med 284: 878–881

Houwert de Jong M H, Bruinse H W, Termijtelen A 1990 The immunology of normal pregnancy and recurrent abortion. Hitten F, Chamberlain G (eds) Clinical physiology in obstetrics. Blackwell Scientific Publications, Oxford, pp 27–38

Huisjes H J 1990a Introduction. Spontaneous abortion: the concept. In: Huisjes H J, Lind T (eds) Clinical obstetrics and gynaecology: early pregnancy failure. Churchill Livingstone, Edinburgh, pp. 1–4

Huisjes H J 1990b Maternal disease and early pregnancy loss. In: Huisjes H J, Lind T (eds) Early pregnancy failure: clinical obstetrics and gynaecology. Churchill Livingstone, Edinburgh, pp 148–153

Imbasciati E, Surian M, Bottin O S et al 1984 Lupus nephropathy and pregnancy. Nephron 36: 46–51

Jansen R P S 1982 Spontaneous abortion incidence in the treatment of infertility. Am J Obstet Gynecol 143: 451–473

Jewlewicz R, Khalaf S, Neuwirth R, Vandewiele R 1976 Obstetric complications after treatment of intrauterine synechiae. Obstet Gynaecol 4: 701–705

Jones G E S, Delfs E 1951 JAMA 146: 121–122

Jones W S 1957 Obstet Gynaecol 10: 113.

Kurt G M 1980 The immune system. In: Hitten F, Chamberlain G (eds) Clinical physiology in obstetrics. Blackwell Scientific Publications, Oxford, pp 101–144

Lauritsen J G 1976 Aetiology of spontaneous abortion: a cytogenetic and epidemiological study of 288 abortuses and their parents. Acta Obstet Gynaecol Scand Suppl 52: 1–29

Lemaire W J, Rice B F, Savard K 1968 Steroid hormone formation of human ovary. V. synthesis of progesterone in vitro in corpo luteal during the reproductive cycle. J Clin Endocrinol Metab 28: 1249–1256

Mowbray J F, Liddle H, Underwood J L et al 1985 Control trial of treatment of recurrent spontaneous abortion by immunisation with paternal cells. Lancet i: 941–943

Murphy H, Lillie E W, Harrison R F 1978 The incompetent cervix in pregnancy. Irish Med J 71: 152–158

Pittaway D E, Karlsten Wentz A 1984 Endometriosis and corpus luteum function: is there a relationship? J Reprod Med 29: 712–716

Prendiville W 1991 HCG for recurrent miscarriage. In: Chalmers I (ed) Oxford data base of perinatal trails. Version 1.D.2. Disc issue 6. Autumn. Record 2890

Regan L 1991 Recurrent miscarriage. Br Med J 302: 543–544

Reinjnders F J L, Thomas C M G et al 1988 Endocrine effects of 17 alpha hydroxy-progesterone caproate during early pregnancy: a double blind clinical trial. Br J Obstet Gynaecol 95: 462–468

Savard K, Marsh J M, Rice V F 1964 Gonadotrophins and ovarian steroidogenesis. Recent Prog Horm Res 21: 285–365

Scheinberg I H, Sternlieb I 1975 Pregnancy in penicillamine-treated patients with Wilson's disease. N Engl J Med 293: 1300–1302

Shearman R F, Garrett W J 1963 A double blind study of the effect of 17-hydroxy-progesterone caproate on abortion rate. Br Med J i: 292–295

Shirodar V W 1955 A method of offered treatment for habitual abortion in the second trimester of pregnancy. Antiseptic 52: 299

Southern P M 1982 Obstet Gynaecol 39: 45

Stirrat G 1983 Recurrent abortion: a review. Br J Obstet Gynaecol 90: 881–883

Stray Pedersen B, Stray Pedersen S 1984 Etiological factors on subsequent reproductive hormones in 195 couples with prior history of habitual abortion. Am J Obstet Gynaecol 148: 140–146

Sunderland C A, Naiem N, Mason J Y, Redman C W J, Stirrat G M 1981 The expression of a major histocompatability antigens by human chorionic villi. J Reprod Immunol 3: 323–331

Taylor C, Falk W P 1981 Prevention of recurrent abortion with leucocyte transfusion. Lancet ii: 68–69

Tho P, Byrd J, McDonagh P 1979 Etiologies and subsequent reproductive performance of 100 couples with recurrent abortion. Fertil Steril 31: 389–395

Trennan P D, McCormack N J, Wojtach A O et al 1978 Immunological studies of the placenta in the systemic lupus erythematosus. Bull Rheum Dis 37: 129–133

Varangot J, Ceder L, Yanotti S 1965 Perfusion of the human placenta in vitro. Am. J Obstet Gynaecol 92: 543–547

Wheler J M, Johnston B M, Malinak L R 1983 Relationship of endometriosis to spontaneous abortion. Fertil Steril 39: 656–660

Yoshimi T, Strot C A, Marshall J R et al 1969 Corpus luteum function in early pregnancy. J Endocrinol 29: 225–230

8

Counselling the infertile patient

B. J. Mostyn

The need to make counselling available to the infertile was first emphasized in the Warnock Inquiry Report of 1984. By the time legislation, resulting from the Inquiry, the Human Fertilization and Embryology Act (HFEA), received the Royal Assent in 1990, requirements for various types of counselling — implications, support and therapeutic — as well as facilities and qualifications for counsellors were carefully defined. Currently the HFEA must not only assess the medical and research aspects of every assisted conception clinic in the UK, but must also assess the counselling facilities available in terms of quality and accessibility.

The original Warnock Inquiry recommended that counselling should be available in every clinic offering infertility treatment; however, the HFEA focuses only on the counselling needs of those in assisted conception clinics. The majority of infertile patients attending outpatient clinics for various types of treatments, excluding assisted conception, are unlikely to have access to counselling or a support group.

The Warnock Inquiry recommendations regarding counselling for the infertile were based on submissions by medical practitioners, social workers, counsellors, religious leaders and the two consumer groups National Association for the Childless (NAC) and CHILD. It became clear to the Inquiry that most patients with an infertility problem experience a special kind of stress — one that is best described as the 'pain of infertility' (Mostyn 1986).

The pain of infertility

Being labelled infertile is devastating to the couple — 'it feels like being given a prison sentence for a crime you did not commit.' For the vast majority of patients infertility is totally unexpected; they look, feel and *act* normally and everything appears to be functioning well. Suddenly young, healthy adults have a medical label, a stigma thrust upon them. The 'one at fault' feels neutered, unattractive, barren, reproductively impotent — 'a freak of nature'. This happens at a time in the life cycle when young adults are building their future — their home, careers, making lifetime friendships, starting a family — and gaining important life experiences and skills — social, travel, DIY,

137

cultural and work-related. Peers are starting their families and talking about how many children to have. The infertile must face the possibility that they may never be parents, never hold their baby in their arms, never be called Mum and Dad, never experience the special love of parent and child and never participate in their children's development. The childless miss out on a normal stage of adult development — parenting.

The infertile experience a deep bereavement over their loss of: a potential child; parenthood; 'a stake in the future'; and self-esteem. To compound their stress they also feel guilty about their experience of grief. They feel that they have not the right to grieve without a 'grief object'. After all they have not actually lost a loved child, they have merely failed to produce one. This phenomenon encouraged NAC's founder, Peter Houghton, to rename the special bereavement experience of infertility 'unfocused grief' (Houghton & Houghton 1987). Unlike their peers, whose lives are regarded as full, even fraught with important family decisions, the infertile feel their lives are frozen owing to the uncertainty about their future — 'Will we or won't we be parents?'

Having accepted the label *infertile* the couple must then seek tests and treatment, which means depending on others for help with the most basic physical function — reproduction. It is not the same as being treated for diabetes, kidney or visual problems, distressing as these may be. The future of one's family, one's genes, one's ancestors are at stake and the infertile can do nothing about it. They feel disempowered. Finding oneself so dependent inevitably brings out their *child* in psychological terms. The infertile feel diminished as adults and their behaviour may often emphasize this feeling. They react like the hurt child who is jealous of others, or the frustrated child who has lost control of the situation, or the angry child who calls out 'It isn't fair!'

Infertility is a life crisis, probably the first crisis that young adults may ever have had to face because experientially infertility is the immovable object. Infertility cannot be solved by persuasion, charm, further education, saving, doing all the right things, knowing the right people, or wealth. As with any other life crisis (divorce, redundancy, etc.) infertility taps into problems from the past and in the present. The most obvious of these is the couple's relationship. However, childhood experiences, especially relations with one's parents, are very likely to come to the fore as well as current relationships with peers, extended family, work colleagues, neighbours and the community. No wonder many infertile people describe themselves as 'coming unstuck' emotionally.

Typical grief reactions

The various symptoms of grieving as first described by C. Murray-Parkes of The Tavistock Institute (Murray-Parkes 1975) are experienced by the infertile, not necessarily in the order described or once only. The majority of patients experience most, if not all, of these symptoms:

- Shock — 'Why me?'
- Sadness — 'What will happen to us?'
- Depression — 'What's the use?'
- Social isolation — 'We are different'
- Loss of self-esteem — 'Only an unworthy person could be fated with this stigma'
- Guilt — 'It was something I did (I didn't do)'
- Shame — 'I've let my family down'
- Anger — The focus is on everything from medical science to parents, doctors to society, family, partner and ultimately oneself
- Fear — Focuses on an empty future.

The counsellor's role is to acknowledge the patient's legitimate grief feelings and thereby give psychological licence (e.g. the right) to grieve over the loss of their fertility. Counselling sessions must focus on exploring the intense and confusing feelings of their grief.

In summary, infertility is a disabling experience, accompanied by physical, social and emotional pain and it strikes people at a stage in their lives when they are least prepared for it. Ideally counselling should be an integral part of every infertility clinic. Not only would the patients be enabled to come to terms with their infertility and dependence on the medical profession in order to found a family, they would be more empowered to seek out/refuse treatment, and to explore alternative ways of parenting or to embrace a childless lifestyle. In addition, when the counsellor becomes part of the medical team in an infertility clinic they are kept up to date on the various tests, drugs and treatments. In turn they create opportunities for the clinical team to gain insights into the normal and typical emotional reactions to infertility. This mutual sharing of disciplines benefits everyone, especially the patients.

RESEARCH STUDY OF INFERTILE COUPLES

An example of the insights that can benefit the medical team resulted from a study by the author which analysed 6 years' experience of counselling infertility outpatients in a large London teaching hospital (The Royal Free) for Professor Robert Shaw's weekly infertility clinic. The aim of the study was to analyse the emotional reactions of typical NHS outpatients to their infertility and to relate these to the cause of the infertility. There were four categories of patients to which couples could be assigned: (1) female problem; (2) male problem; (3) unexplained infertility; and (4) both partners with a problem.

Previous research has examined the wide range of emotional reactions to infertility generally, such as feelings of anger and grief as well as fear of loss of control over one's life (Rosenfeld & Mitchell 1979). Others have shown that anxiety scores increased as the length of time for investigations and treatment was extended and uncertainty about the future grew (Edelmann & Golombok 1989, Bell 1981, Humphrey 1984, Dennerstein & Morse 1985).

The specific hypothesis to be tested was that emotional responses to infertility vary by *cause* of infertility. More than 450 individuals were seen over a 6-year period (1985–1991) by the author–counsellor. Patients were self-selected (they asked to see a counsellor) or were selected by the medical team. The majority were seen at least twice, some as often as 12 or 13 times. Two-thirds were seen with their partners at least once, and each session lasted approximately 1 hour. Case notes were made after each session; many of the notes included direct quotes, as well as an analysis of the emotional state of the patients.

From all of the patients seen, 192 couples were chosen for inclusion in the study. Those eliminated were either involved in other research at the Royal Free Hospital, or had to be eliminated owing to language difficulties. The age range of the patients in the study was very broad — 19–54 — with a median of 34 years (Table 8.1).

When the cause of the infertility was analysed, the most common problems were tubal for women and low sperm counts for men; the next most common were miscarriage/stillbirth/ectopic for women and azoospermia for men. Where patients had unexplained infertility one-third had experienced secondary infertility, and 17% had recently experienced an associated medical problem (Table 8.2).

The type of infertility problem experienced, e.g. male, female, unexplained or 'both with a problem', appeared to produce a different pattern of emotional responses. When the cause of the problem was female infertility, the women seemed caught up in a terrible emotional triangle of guilt–fear–anger, with

Table 8.1   Characteristics of the sample by cause of infertility (*n* = 192 couples)

Cause of infertility	% of sample	Age at first visit: range and median	Partner came at least once (%)	Childless partnership (%)	Number of times seen by counsellor: range and mean
Female *n* = 57	30	R = 19–43 M = 32.5 (females)	37	77	R = 1–12 M = 2.4
Male *n* = 55	29	R = 24–54 M = 35 (males)	86	80	R = 1–7 M = 2.0
Unexplained *n* = 58	30	R = 22–49 M = 34 (males and females)	69	71	R = 1–7 M = 2.0
Both *n* = 22	11	R = 21–46 M = 35 (males and females)	86	86	R = 1–13 M = 2.0
n = 192	100%	R = 19–54 M = 34	Av. 66%	Av. 77%	R = 1–13 M = 2.0

Table 8.2 Nature of the infertility problem by cause (n = 192 couples)

Female problem n = 57	%	Male problem n = 55	%	Both with a problem n = 22 His	%	Hers	%
Tubal	44	Low sperm count	44	Low count	64	Tubal	32
Miscarriage, stillbirth, ectopic	18	Azoospermia	18	Impotence	14	Ovulatory	27
Ovulatory	16	Vasectomy reversal partial success	11	Poor-quality sperm	5	Miscarriage	14
				Antibodies	5	Fibroids/ adhesions	14
Endometriosis	11	Low motility	7	Azoospermia	5	Mucous hostility	9
Early ovarian failure	7	Impotence	7	Low motility	4	Chromosomal abnormality	4
Mucous hostility	3	Poor-quality sperm	5	Chromosomal abnormality	4		
Hormone imbalance (following mastectomy)		Antibodies	5				
	3	Retroactive ejaculation	2				
	100%		99%		100%		100%

Unexplained infertility n = 58	%
Secondary infertility	33
Fairly serious medical problem: TB, meningitis, thryoid, etc.	17
3 years or more infertility treatments	9
Others	41
	100%

each emotion feeding the other to the point where they felt there was no way out — 'I feel caught in a web.' When male infertility was diagnosed, the men experienced a terrible shock and typically reacted with resignation to their perceived new status as one of life's victims, rather than the masters of their own lives. A label of 'unexplained infertility' created feelings of uncertainty, anxiety and of self-doubt about many areas of what they perceived as their 'thwarted' lives. The 'double jeopardy' scenario, where neither one is normally fertile, created feelings of despair, hopelessness, 'emptiness' and an intense fear of the future. The *dominant* emotion expressed by the patient(s) analysed by cause of the infertility problem is shown in Table 8.3. Patients obviously experience a mixture of emotions. However, one emotion tended to dominate and this emotion persisted over time. The other emotions which 'shadowed' the dominant one also showed stability over time. For example, depression and anger accompanied anxiety in the 'unexplained' group.

Table 8.3 Dominant emotional response by cause of infertility (n = 192 couples)

Female[a] n = 57	%	Male[b] n = 55	%	Unexplained n = 58	%	Both n = 22	%
Guilt	26	Depression	22	Anxiety	40	Depression	36
Fear	21	Guilt	20	Depression	20	Anger	18
Anger	12	Shock	15	Anger	14	Anxiety	14
Anxiety	11	Conflicted/ confused	11	Fear	10	Fear	9
Depression	7	Grief	9	Isolation	5	Conflicted/ Confused	9
Grief	7	Anger	9	Conflicted/ confused	3	Relief—shared problem is better	9
Shock	7						
Isolation	5	Fear	5	Guilt	3		
Determined to go on	4	Determined to 'win'	5	Determined to go on	3		
		Anxiety	4	Obsessed with problem	2	Guilt	5
	100%		100%		100%		100%

[a]Women's feelings only.
[b]Men's feelings only (14% of cases, as reported by partner who was the only one to come for counselling).

These intense emotional experiences were typical for the type of infertility problem regardless of the presence of children from a previous or current partnership. Thus the experience of secondary infertility seemed to tap into the same deep, basic emotions as primary infertility. The fact that the type of infertility problem makes patients more susceptible to certain emotional reactions has important implications, not only for the way in which the counsellor perceives and approaches the patient, but also for the way medical staff prepare themselves to deal with the emotional as well as the physical problems. From the study four psychological types of patients have emerged. Each one will be described, with quotes to exemplify the types of feelings expressed.

The female burden

Women with an infertility problem are typically caught up in a terrible emotional triangle of *guilt* — 'What did I do?' *fear* — 'What will become of me?' and *anger* — 'It isn't fair!'. Each emotion reinforces the other.

Guilt

Guilt is the principal component (see Table 8.3). Women with an infertility problem are more likely to blame themselves than attribute their problem to 'bad luck', the stresses of modern life or bad medical treatment, although these reasons are often mentioned as well. They dredge up from their past everything which they did, or failed to do, that could have caused their problem.

> 'My own social life was the cause of my problem; the swinging sixties and the sexual revolution are getting their own back.'

> 'It is my own fault. Years ago I gave into an abortion.'

> 'Eating badly, going on crash diets, casual affairs, wearing Tampax, no wonder I've got blocked tubes.'

Their infertility becomes a punishment for past transgressions. To add to their emotional burden, it is not uncommon for women to experience feelings of guilt when their partner is the infertile one! Connolly et al (1987) also found that when there is a male fertility problem both partners feel guilty.

> 'It's odd, I feel guilty that it's not me; sounds crazy really.'

> 'I feel such a failure; he has three kids by his first marriage and I really want his child but his reversal was not a success.'

Fear

The burden of infertility and accompanying strong guilt reactions unleashes feelings of fear about an unknown future. Old anxieties and fears are aroused as well; fears of being burdened with an imperfect body; fears of losing control over their lives; fears of tempting fate (a fate which has decided that she should be childless).

> 'My mother always said that because I had irregular periods I would have trouble having children.'

> 'It was my mother and the GP who decided I should have the abortion; no one ever asked me. Now it's the same all over again, being in treatment — somebody else is always in charge of your life.'

> 'Now that we are on the IVF waiting list I feel that we are going too far trying to have our own child and we may end up with a handicapped child.'

Anger

Intense fear and feelings of guilt inevitably arouse feelings of anger. Most typically that anger is directed towards feelings of helplessness, the unfairness of infertility, insensitive or inconsistent treatment, one's worthless self, or the unsupportive partner.

> 'If this treatment doesn't work I don't know what I will do; I can't imagine life without children.'

> 'It's so unfair; there are all these people who have abortions, it's all wrong.'

'We have a poor PCT; one doctor says ignore it, another says it's not a good sign; I feel thrown around.'

'I feel so worthless, what have I done to deserve this!' (Early ovarian failure)

'It may be hopeless, and he's not a strength to me. I can't talk to him about it, he's so closed off.'

Women's feelings of anger and fear are exacerbated by the fact that they are less likely to be supported by their partners when they have the infertility problem. In this sample women were accompanied by their partners in only 37% of cases, while 86% of women attended when their partner had the problem. Women who attend the clinic and come to see the counsellor on their own feel isolated and acutely in need of someone to share the burden. During the 6 years of counselling reported here, two-thirds of counselling time was spent with women on their own. Other researchers have also found that the primary reason for women seeking counselling was feelings of isolation (Connolly et al 1987).

In summary, infertility is devastating for most women, whether the primary cause of the problem is female, male or both have a problem. It is probably her first life crisis and she realizes how many fears she actually has, the intensity of her anger and resentment towards life, her partner, and more importantly, herself as emphasized by her strong guilt reactions. Freeman et al (1985) found 50% of women reported that being labelled infertile was the most upsetting experience of their lives.

'It's hard to bear, I wouldn't wish this on anybody.'

Since female infertility is a major life crisis, counselling must aim to help women explore their fears and own their feelings, especially guilt and anger which evolve around their infertility. There is also a need to explore other aspects of their lives that also seem to have fallen apart with the crisis of infertility — career/job, family and social relationships. When the male partner is the focus for anger and guilt and she experiences him as unsupportive, there is a need to focus the counselling sessions on the relationship — strengths, weaknesses, hopes and fears for the future, what attracted them to each other, what will keep the relationship going, and what might tear it apart. Preferably these issues should be confronted by both partners. However, the reluctance of many men to become involved with both treatment and counselling when there is a female problem means that these issues are often only explored with the woman. The counselling skills most essential for women with an infertility problem are those from crisis counselling and marriage guidance.

Male resignation

Because the diagnosis of male infertility is so unexpected, the most typical male response is to feel victimized and depressed. The shock of discovering that he is not *normal* changes his self image. No longer is he the master of his life, he is the victim of circumstances. This is not surprising, since the vast majority of men and women attending an infertility clinic do not suspect that there could be anything wrong on the male side. Like most people, they assume that infertility is a 'female problem'. It is a devastating shock to be told that one has no, few, deformed or nearly immobile sperm, or that one's chances of fathering a child are 'next to nil'. Add to this the fact that they are usually informed that there is little or no treatment for male problems, and the emotional responses of depression, hopelessness, shock and guilt, as well as resignation, on the part of men is understandable.

Depression

Men tend to talk about feeling 'gutted', 'shattered' or 'destroyed' when they first find out they are the reason for the infertility. Many find it just as difficult to accept a year or so later.

> 'Ever since we found out I've been depressed and so has J. We break down every so often. We just can't help it.'

Unfortunately for some men their infertility reinforces an existing poor self image because it represents yet another area of their life where they feel the victim and not the master.

> 'It's another area of my life I'm not in charge of, like my work, our flat, our social life.'

> 'I always feared it would be me, another part of my insecurity.'

Guilt

Feelings of depression and despair are typically accompanied by guilt towards the partner and feelings of insecurity in the relationship. His feeling that he has ruined her chances of becoming a mother, especially if she is particularly maternal, is a great source of pain to him.

> 'I crack every so often when I think about it, that it's me preventing us having a family.'

> 'I just feel so inadequate in the relationship now.'

> 'I can't see the marriage lasting without children; she is a born mother.'

Shock

The way in which the man and his partner are presented with the news of his infertility will often influence the extent to which he will feel shocked and numb.

'The consultant at the other hospital said to my wife "You better find another man, your husband won't give you children, his sperm are too deformed!" I was stunned for days.'

The registrar just looked up and said "From your tests you had better consider AID or adoption", and then he suggested we get information from you. I don't know what to say or what to do.'

'I phoned up and was told there was no hope of us having children together. I don't know how I got home, or when I told her; I can't remember anything.'

While the typical reaction to male infertility is resignation, characterized by depression or despair and guilt as the man tries to come to terms with the shock, a small group — those in a second marriage who already have children and are infertile because of a failed vasectomy reversal — react with determination to solve the problem. They see their infertility as a challenge, a problem to be conquered. Instead of feeling victims they feel they are the masters of the situation.

'The reversal wasn't a success but that doesn't mean we can't have a family. I feel determined to succeed and I'm set on AID — it's more natural.'

Unfortunately, not all of the partners are ready to consider alternative ways of founding a family so readily, especially if she has never had children.

In summary, male infertility is so unexpected, so hopeless in terms of current treatment options, for the majority of men that it creates an unexpected grief reaction with accompanying despair, as well as feelings of guilt that they are preventing their partner from founding a family. Self-esteem and confidence plummet.

Bereavement counselling is essential for these men and their partners, who have indeed lost something; a stake in the future; the symbolic loss of their manhood/adulthood; and the possibility of becoming a parent. The various stages of grief need to be worked through with psychological licence given to cry, rage and face one's worst fears, including the fact that the marriage may not last.

Thwarted lives: unexplained infertility

The label of *unexplained infertility* creates feeling of uncertainty, instability and self-doubt among infertile couples. The relationship inevitably suffers. Daniluk (1988) found that couples with unexplained infertility experienced the highest dissatisfaction with their marital and sexual relationships. This is understandable; when no explanation for the failure to conceive can be found, there is bound to be doubt, speculation and uncertainty — 'Is it you?', 'Is it me?' 'Is it both of us?' Emotional reactions of guilt, fear and distrust between partners are inevitable.

'Deep down I'm afraid it's me and she's afraid it's her. At the same time we both feel it could be the other one; it doesn't help the relationship at all.'

Living with uncertainty concerning such an important issue — 'Will we or won't we be parents?' — creates a life crisis which can permeate every facet of life, including work, friendships, relationships with the family/community, etc.

> 'The uncertainty is terrible; our lives have been frozen for more than five years now.'

Lives become frozen because major decisions are postponed until the outcome of the infertility tests and treatment are known. Plans for the future are replaced by fears of the future. Understandably, anxiety and frustration are the dominant feelings amongst this group of patients. These feelings are accompanied by the realization that they cannot get on and plan their future like their contemporaries, which also arouses strong emotions of depression, social isolation and, ultimately, anger.

Anxiety

Being labelled *unexplained* in an age which is geared up to technological advances and efficiency, with explanations for nearly everything, is hard to accept. Men and women look for their own explanations and possible solutions. Many become obsessed with the subject of their infertility. They examine every aspect of their lives, past and present, seeking the cause of the 'problem'. They worry over past 'mistakes' in lifestyle: diet, experiments with drugs, too many partners, the pill/coil, previous illnesses or accidents, emotional crises, participation in strenuous, sports, dance or exercise, etc.

Bus drivers and travelling reps express concern about sitting all day and decreasing their sperm counts. (Couples with unexplained infertility are more likely to read *everything* they can get their hands on relating to infertility.) Women from close-knit families have the added pressure of getting 'advice' from various family members on how to increase their fertility, which ranges from giving up the stress of a job, to getting a job to take your mind off it; from advice to drink certain teas, to stop drinking tea and coffee; and from not eating meat, to stir-frying everything, etc.

> 'It's the uncertainty that's hard to bear; I can't see a future.'

> 'Everything I do worries me, one cigarette, one drink, even what I am thinking — will it mean less of a chance of conceiving?'

Depression

The two major subgroups amongst those with *unexplained infertility* — those with secondary infertility (33% in this study) and those where one partner has an ongoing or recent serious medical problem (meningitis, thyroid, blood pressure, epilepsy, etc.; 17%) — were particularly fearful and depressed about the future.

'I dread getting up in the morning and facing the emptiness, we just ache for children.'

'It's so depressing to feel outcasts in the family.'

'We feel such failures, all our friends are on their second or third child now, and she keeps asking for a brother or sister.'

Some of the women with medical problems fear they might actually be blocking a pregnancy because they have some anxiety about coping with childbearing, or that pregnancy could make their problem worse, or they might have a handicapped child. This makes them all the more depressed about life.

'It's probably me preventing the pregnancy. My mother developed MS after she had me.'

'I'm scared of more tests, scared of what I might find out — that there is something serious that's wrong.'

'I've had a lot of problems and I know I couldn't cope with a handicapped child. Maybe we should give up trying.' (Epileptic)

Anger

With no explanation for their infertility, with other medical problems creating anxiety and, for some, being in treatment a long time (9%, 3 years or more), it is not surprising that many couples with unexplained infertility come to the conclusion that they have been treated unfairly by fate. They then feel very angry.

'We've been in treatment for eight years, and nothing; we have nothing. It's so unfair!'

'I sometimes feel there is a curse on me. Why should I be punished this way? I've always been good to everyone.'

In summary, couples with *unexplained infertility* feel thwarted in their attempt to overcome their infertility, since no reason can be found for it. To add to their stress, many may have been able to conceive a first child easily. For them their infertility is even more of a mystery, or a curse. Having another serious medical problem further enhances their feelings of inadequacy. Support counselling is essential. Just being there and encouraging them to express their frustration, anxiety, anger and fear, as well as acknowledge how they are feeling, will be reassuring, particularly when they can accept that these are normal feelings. Daniluk (1988) found that many couples with unexplained infertility indicated a desire for counselling just to know if they were 'normal'. Psychosexual counselling may be essential for those who fear they are 'not doing it right'. However, for most 'person-centred' counselling should be the main approach, which focuses on empowering the couple to help themselves by discovering the positive things in their lives and in themselves.

Double jeopardy: both partners have a problem

Faced with the realization that neither partner is fertile, couples experience a depressive powerlessness which makes them feel angry at everything in life and anxious about the future.

Depression

When both have been labelled infertile, life feels 'suspended' and 'empty'. Sadly, for many it is a reconfirmation that they have always been unlucky; they are life's 'losers'.

> 'My sister was always brighter and prettier and she has two children. I'm 38 now. We have little chance, I'm a failure again.'

> 'My work, now this, I feel washed up on the shore.'

Anger

A feeling of being doubly unlucky generates angry feelings towards nearly everything: medical science and doctors for letting them down; society for being insensitive; friends and neighbours for being so fertile; each other (who remind one of the 'problem'); and towards themselves. Not infrequently wives accuse husbands of not trying to find a solution, typically within alternative medicine. Husbands accuse partners of having unrealistic hopes after so many failures with treatments. The relationship can deteriorate into childish game-playing, even during counselling sessions.

> 'You keep saying it's me, what about your low sperm count?' 'Well I don't have any endometriosis do I?'

> 'I think it's just time to stop trying I could be content as we are, but you want to go on having miscarriages!'

Fears of the future are so threatening that strong aggressive feelings may be provoked.

> 'I can't get near my friends with babies, I fear I will take one. I'm like a volcano about to explode.'

> I'm just sure something really serious is wrong and they just aren't finding it, so our lives will always be a question mark.'

Anxiety

When neither is totally sterile, the anxiety and fear of the future creates a dilemma — should they give up tests and treatment, or hang on to the one shred of hope they have and persevere? Those who have had one or more failed attempts at IVF (15% of the sample) felt particularly torn between going on and perhaps 'overcoming the odds', or facing the painful loss of yet another failure.

'I don't know what we should do. I have this feeling of wanting to be rescued.'

'I feel so incomplete after a failed IVF. It's like a baby's been lost!'

In summary, when both partners have a fertility problem, intense feelings of helplessness and powerlessness take over. They relive the frustrations and despair of powerless children, reacting childishly with temper tantrums, resentment towards authority, sulks and self-pity.

'It's you!' 'No, it's you!'

'I'm really upset, it's so unfair. Just because his kids live with us we can't have IVF.'

'Why do I bother to come along, no one talks to me, examines me or offers any treatment or any more tests.' (Male)

Couples caught in *double jeopardy* tend to revert to what the transactional analyst calls the 'child ego state'. Unfortunately, many of them withdraw from decision making altogether and continue to come to the clinic in the hope of being rescued by a miracle or new scientific breakthrough. This reaction to a serious problem is what transaction analysis calls the 'waiting for Father Christmas syndrome'. They want to believe that, like all good stories, it will end happily.

These couples require counselling together and separately in order to air their fears, anger, depression and resentments. It is important that the counsellor makes sure they 'hear' and acknowledge the intensity of the feelings they express. Transactional analysis focuses on helping the patient accept their destructive, childish reactions to their infertility and to discover how many 'childish tapes' they continue to replay when they face stress in any facet of their lives. Double jeopardy couples need to be challenged to take responsibility for creating their own future — a new beginning — once they come to terms with the fact that they are *not* going to be rescued. They need to explore their personal and collective strengths and abilities and to rediscover all they have to offer each other, themselves and society — vocationally, socially, emotionally and practically. In other words, they need help learning to *like* themselves again.

CONCLUSIONS

For the vast majority of patients infertility is an unexpected life crisis which creates anxiety, emotional distress, strains in the relationship and loss of confidence. This chapter has examined how patients *experience* their infertility as they describe and express it verbally and non-verbally in a counselling context. The results presented, which were based on case notes by the author–counsellor, have been analysed by *cause* of infertility in order to provide insights into the psychology of infertility and the implications for the way in which the counsellor should approach the patient/couple.

The findings from this qualitative investigation among 192 couples is that the *type* of infertility problem experienced, including unexplained, taps into certain specific emotional responses. For instance, when women 'are the problem', they experience a major life crisis; they become caught up in an emotional triangle of guilt–fear–anger ('What did I do?' 'What will become of me?' 'It isn't fair!'). Their distress is often exacerbated by the fact that typically they have no support from their partner. These women will benefit most from a combination of crisis and marriage guidance counselling.

When men are 'the problem', they experience grief for themselves and guilt regarding their partners, which is often made worse by the partner's loyalty. For many it will be the first time in their lives that they will experience themselves as victims, rather than masters over their lives. Bereavement counselling is essential for these men who have indeed lost something important – a stake in the future, as well as a symbolic loss of manhood.

Those whose infertility remains unexplained experience fear and anxiety about a future they cannot control. They perceive their lives as thwarted, especially those with secondary infertility. These couples benefit most from person-centred counselling, often augmented by psychosexual counselling, when they need the reassurance that they are 'normal'.

When both partners have a problem, there is a tendency for at least one, if not both, to revert to the 'child ego state' triggered by feelings of helplessness, which they express as anger, self-pity, distrust of authority and fantasies of 'waiting to be rescued'. Counselling needs to be based on transactional analysis to help them explore their destructive child's emotional reactions to the problem, and work towards getting in touch with their adult self, by taking control of their own lives, planning for the future and accepting that they will not be rescued.

ACKNOWLEDGEMENTS

My thanks to Professor Peter Braude for helpful comments and suggestions and to Mrs Eva Goldhagen for her patience in preparing the manuscript.

REFERENCES

Bell J S 1981 Psychological problems among patients attending an infertility clinic. J Psychosom Res 25: 1–3

Connolly K J, Edelmann R J, Cooke I D 1987 Distress and marital problems associated with infertility. J. Reprod Infant Psychol 5: 49–57

Daniluk J C 1988 Infertility: intrapersonal and interpersonal impact. Fertil Steril 49: 982–990

Dennerstein L, Morse C 1985 Psychological Issues in IVF clinics. Obstet Gynaecol 12: 835–846

Edelmann R J, Golombok S 1989 Stress and reproductive failure. J Reprod Infant Psychol 7: 79–86

Freeman E W, Boxer A S, Rickels K et al 1985 Psychological evaluation and support in a program of IVF and embryo transfer. Fertil Steril 43: 48–53

Houghton D, Houghton P 1987 Coping with childlessness. Allen and Unwin, London
Humphrey M 1984 Infertility and alternative parenting. In: Broome A, Wallace L M (eds)
    Gynaecological problems. Tavistock, London
Mostyn B 1986 The patient's point of view. Irish J Med Sci 155: 9–11
Murray-Parkes C 1975 Bereavement: studies of grief in adult life. Penguin, London
Rosenfeld D L Mitchell E 1979 Treating the emotional aspects of infertility: counselling
    services in an infertility clinic. Am J Obstet Gynaecol 22: 255–267

Gynaecology

9

Cervical screening and teenage women

P. I. Blomfield   I. D. Duncan

Cervical screening programmes aim to reduce deaths from cervical cancer. In those countries operating successful programmes, the majority of those who develop and die from cervical cancer are older women who have never participated in a screening programme. Opportunistic screening has meant that the bulk of smears have been taken in younger women in whom cervical intra-epithelial neoplasia (CIN) is more prevalent. This means that some very young women, i.e. teenagers, have also been screened and the question must be asked whether or not these women are truly likely to benefit.

CURRENT RECOMMENDATIONS

National recommendations for cervical screening programmes have varied. In 1974 the Walton Report suggested commencing screening from the age of 18 onwards. The International Agency for Research on Cancer examined ten screening programmes, suggesting anticipated percentage falls in the incidence of cervical cancer with smears of various frequencies in various age groups. They concluded that 5-yearly screening of women aged between 20 and 64 years should reduce the incidence by 84%, whilst 3-yearly screening of the same age group would improve the reduction further to 91%. The DHSS and the Scottish Home and Health Department in 1987 advocated screening from 20 years, at least 5-yearly. The Intercollegiate Working Party Report published by the Royal College of Obstetricians and Gynaecologists (RCOG) in 1987 strongly supported computerized call and recall of women from the age of 20 years. Opportunistic screening has still been carried out upon teenagers.

PREVALENCE OF CYTOLOGICAL AND HISTOLOGICAL ABNORMALITY IN TEENAGE POPULATIONS

There is no doubt that cervical abnormalities can be detected in teenagers by cervical cytology. Table 9.1 describes prevalence rates of cytological abnormality and histologically confirmed CIN III or carcinoma in situ (CIS) in several different teenage populations. MacGregor & Teper (1978) reported on

Table 9.1   Comparison of prevalence rates of cytological abnormality and CIS/CIN III in teenage populations and samples

Study	Sample size	Age group	Prevalence of cytological abnormality (Rate per 1000)	Prevalence of CIS/CIN III (Rate per 1000)
MacGregor & Teper (1978) Scotland	9004	<20	16	1.8
Sadeghi et al (1984) California	194 069	15–19	53	2.6
Zaninetti et al (1986) Milan	2024	<20	62	1.0
(1990) Birmingham, unpublished data	1163	15–19	142 (71[a])	3.4
Mitchel & Medley (1988) Victoria	46 342	<20	43[a]	1.1[b]

[a]Prevalence of cytological abnormality from 1980 to 1987 in teenagers in Victoria.
[b]Estimated prevalence from years 1985 and 1986 of teenagers in Victoria.
[c]Prevalence of cytological abnormality, and of dyskaryotic smears.

the prevalence of cytological abnormality in over 9000 women under the age of 20 between 1967 and 1976. The frequency of atypical cytology in this population increased from 11 per 1000 in 1967 to 19 per 1000 in 1976. However, only 1.8 per 1000 screened progressed to CIS in the follow-up period, while 0.3 per 1000 were treated for lower-grade lesions. More recent publications from different centres show an even higher rate of cytological abnormality, but the amount of CIN III detected remains similar and represents only a very small proportion of the whole.

Most of the cytological abnormalities seen in these young populations are minor and often transient. Indeed, in the observational study by MacGregor & Teper (1978) over 60% regressed spontaneously to normal. Most of the lesions demonstrated in teenagers reflect low-grade disease, either human papilloma viral change or CIN I. It is theoretically possible to distinguish between these two conditions (Fox & Buckley 1990), but in practical terms they are not robust diagnoses and are prone to both inter- and intra-observer variation (Robertson et al 1989). The significance of low-grade disease in terms of the natural history of cervical neoplasia is unclear and it is possible that the abnormality being detected in these teenagers reflects an infectious rather than neoplastic process. Teenagers embarking upon sexual activity but not as yet settled with one partner are prone to various sexually transmitted diseases, including human papillomavirus infection. Nevertheless, the higher grades of CIN are sometimes encountered when teenagers with abnormal smears are investigated.

Zaninetti et al (1986) investigated risk factors for cytological abnormality in 2097 teenagers in Milan; 126 (6%) were referred for colposcopy because of cytological abnormality. Only 11 subjects had histological evidence of CIN II and 2 of CIN III. In an unpublished study of 1219 Birmingham teenagers examined between 1988 and 1990, the vast majority of 170 abnormal smears showed either borderline (52.3%) or mildly dyskaryotic (47%) changes. More than half of these subjects had histological evidence of human papillomavirus infection without CIN. Colposcopically directed punch biopsy confirmed CIN II in only 1 of the 88 subjects with borderline changes, and 5 of the 76 subjects with dyskaryosis. CIN III was not found in any of those with borderline cytology but was demonstrated in 5 of those with dyskaryosis. These rates of cervical intra-epithelial neoplasia are much lower than comparative prospective studies of subjects with mildly dyskaryotic smears (see Table 9.2) and reflect the differences in the age groups of the populations examined.

Other authors have reported higher rates of CIN II and CIN III in teenagers referred for colposcopic assessment. These are, however, highly selected populations. Walker et al (1990) found 10 cases of CIN II and 9 cases of CIN III in 44 teenagers referred with mild cytological abnormality. Haddad et al (1988) found 36 cases of CIN II and 29 of CIN III in 96 teenagers referred with a suspicious smear, but this group may well have contained women with moderate dyskaryosis. Undoubtedly, higher grade CIN does occur to some extent in teenagers but there is good evidence from population-based studies that despite high rates of minor cytological abnormality only a very small proportion will have high grade intra-epithelial

Table 9.2 Comparison of prevalence rates of CIN for teenagers with cytological abnormality with prospective studies of women with similar cytological abnormalities, but of older age groups

Study	Sample	Age (years)	% CIN I	% CIN II	% CIN III
Older age groups					
Giles et al (1989) (single mildly dyskaryotic smear)	143	29 (mean)	21.6	14.0	17.5
Giles et al (1989) (<6 months since mildly dyskaryotic smear)	121	29 (mean)	20.6	16.5	19.0
Luesley et al (unpublished) (referral smear mildly dyskaryotic)[a]	337	29 (mean)	21.4	15.7	26.1
Teenage populations					
Birmingham (1990) Atypical cytology (not graded as dyskaryotic)	88	15–19	13.6	1.1	0.0
Birmingham (1990) Dyskaryotic cytology (majority mild dyskaryosis)	76	15–19	17.1	6.6	6.6
Zaninetti et al (1986) Cytological evidence of CIN	110	15–19	78.0[b]	10	1.8

[a]Data from LLETZ database, Dudley Road Hospital, Birmingham. Women of 20 years and over referred with mild dyskaryosis for colposcopic assessment.
[b]This group did not differentiate between CIN I and human papillomavirus infection.

neoplasia. There is certainly no justification for routine screening of teenagers if the lesion is likely to be detected at a later date before invasion has occurred. Fortunately, invasive cervical cancer is extremely uncommon in the teenage population. In 1984 in England and Wales the incidence was 2 per million and no teenagers died from this disease.

TREATMENT OF TEENAGERS WITH CIN

Cervical screening programmes do have a debit side. Although the test is acceptable to most women, by and large it is not one to which they look forward. An abnormal smear report is met with alarm and despondency, usually unjustified and entirely out of proportion to the degree of abnormality present. Further anxieties are engendered in those referred for colposcopy and treatment (Wilkinson et al 1990, Lerman et al 1991, Posner & Vessey 1988, Campion et al 1988).

Modern treatments are aimed at the eradication of CIN while conserving cervical function. In teenagers, the squamocolumnar junction is almost always clearly visible because of cervical eversion induced by adolescent oestrogen surges. This means colposcopic diagnosis is normally satisfactory and the clinician can choose from a range of destructive or excisional methods of treatment, once a diagnosis is confirmed. In the knowledge that a significant proportion of lower-grade lesions will regress spontaneously, there may be an argument for conservative management by observation in this young age group, provided follow-up can be ensured. Neither electrocoagulation diathermy, cold coagulation, laser vaporization, cryosurgery nor loop diathermy excision have been associated with subsequent cervical incompetence. Hillard et al (1991) did observe a 9% incidence of pelvic inflammatory disease in a group of adolescents undergoing cryotherapy for CIN and recommended aggressive preventive measures for such complications. This could result in infertility which would be particularly disastrous in this age group, who may not as yet have embarked on childbearing. Such an outcome following treatment for an asymptomatic lesion possibly destined to regress spontaneously is highly undesirable.

IDENTIFICATION OF TEENAGERS AT HIGH RISK OF DEVELOPING CYTOLOGICAL ABNORMALITY

The question has to be asked whether it is possible to identify a high risk group of teenagers who would warrant screening. Walker et al (1990) studied the obstetric histories of 100 teenagers undergoing cervical biopsy. Ten of these patients had been referred with vulval warts and 90 with abnormal cytology. CIN was present in 51 women and absent in 49. There was no difference in the distribution of pregnancies in the CIN and non-CIN groups. Nulliparity or a history of abortion was commoner in both teenage groups than was a history of childbearing. Thus, the obstetric history was of no value in predicting those who were likely to have CIN. In the Birmingham study referred to above, 1163 young women were recruited consecutively from a family planning clinic in an attempt to predict cytological abnormality on the basis of known risk factors for disease. A detailed questionnaire was used to collect information on the following variables: age, social status, past medical and obstetric history, smoking and alcohol habits, sexually transmitted diseases, genital warts and a detailed sexual history. Both univariate and stepwise discriminant analysis were used to compare data from those with abnormal cytology with the data collected from those with normal cytology. Five factors were identified as predictors for abnormal smears using discriminant analysis: history of infection or exposure to genital warts, alcohol consumption, number of sexual partners, age of the first sexual partner, and STD clinic attendance. However, using this information to try to predict subjects with abnormal smears, only 10% of subjects found to have actual cytological abnormality would have been detected. Further analyses were carried out to try to predict those subjects with CIN, from amongst those with cytological abnormality. The risk factors identified would have predicted only 24% of those with CIN. In conclusion, a high-risk group of teenagers cannot be predicted or selected despite the availability of detailed information relating to sexual and other risk factors.

CONCLUSION

A working party of the National Health Service Cervical Screening Programme Coordinating Network recently came to the conclusion that the incidence of invasive carcinoma of the cervix does not justify including women under the age of 20 in the national call and recall system, provided there is good compliance with the programme in the early 20s age range (Duncan 1992). This does not mean that cervical smears should not be taken in teenagers. Smears may still be employed as a diagnostic test in individual cases but routine screening should be deferred until the age of 20. Those women who have not become sexually active by this age are likely to decline their initial invitation to attend for screening. Their introduction to screening may be on an opportunistic basis while attending for contraceptive or antenatal advice.

Current opinion is that teenagers stand to lose more than they would gain from cytological screening for CIN.

KEY POINTS FOR CLINICAL PRACTICE

1. Routine inclusion of teenagers in screening programmes is not justified upon present evidence, assuming good compliance after the age of 20 years.

2. Smears may still be employed as a diagnostic test in individual cases; however, the identification of 'high risk' teenagers using current knowledge of risk factors for CIN is unlikely to yield high returns.

3. Current treatment modalities for cervical intra-epithelial neoplasia are suitable for teenagers with established disease. However, there is a case for conservative management in those with low grade disease, since regression rates are likely to be high.

REFERENCES

Brinton L A, Hamman R F, Huggins G R et al 1987 Sexual and reproductive factors for invasive squamous cell cervical cancer. J Natl Cancer Inst 79: 23–30

Campion M J, Brown J R, McCance D J et al 1988 Psychological trauma of an abnormal cervical smear. Br J Obstet Gynaecol 95: 175–181

Department of Health and Social Security 1984 Health Services Development. Screening for cervical cancer. DHSS, London, (HC84(17))

Duncan I D (ed) 1992 National Health Service Cervical Screening Programme, National Coordinating Network. Guidelines for clinical practice and programme management

Fox H, Buckley C H 1990 Current problems in the pathology of intraepithelial lesions of the uterine cervix. Histopathology. 17: 1–6

Giles J A, Deery A, Crow J et al 1989 The accuracy of repeat cytology in women with mildly dyskaryotic smears. Br J Obstet Gynaecol 96: 1067–1070

Haddad N G, Hussein I Y, Livingstone J R B et al 1988 Colposcopy in teenagers. Br Med J 297: 29–30

Hillard P A, Biro FM, Wildey L 1991 Complications of cervical cryotherapy in adolescents. J Reprod Med 36: 711–716

IARC Working group on evaluation of cervical screening programmes 1986 Screening for squamous cervical cancer: duration of low risk after negative results of cervical cytology and its implications for screening policies. Br Med J 293: 659–664

Intercollegiate working party on cervical cytology screening 1987 Report. Royal College of Obstetricians and Gynaecologists, London, p 8

Lerman C, Miller S M, Scarborough R et al 1991 Adverse psychological consequences of positive cytologic cervical screening. Am J Obstet Gynecol 165: 658–662

MacGregor J E, Teper S 1978 Uterine cervical cytology and young women. Lancet i: 1029–1031

Mitchell H, Medley G 1988 Pap smear results of Victorian teenagers, 1980–1987. Aust NZ J Obstet Gynaecol 28: 213–215

Posner T, Vessey M 1988 Psychosexual trauma of an abnormal cervical smear. Br J Obstet Gynaecol 95: 729

Report by ad hoc Group of the Histopathology Sub-Committee of the Scientific Services Advisory Group on the Cervical Cytology Service in Scotland 1987

Report of the task force appointed by the Conference of Deputy Ministers of Health — the Walton Report 1976 Cervical Cancer Screening Programmes. Can Med Assoc 114: 1003–1033

Robertson A J, Anderson J M, Swanson Beck J et al 1989 Observer variability in histopathological reporting of cervical biopsy specimens. J Clin Pathol 42: 231–238

Sadeghi S B, Hsieh E W, Gunn S W 1984 Prevalence of cervical intraepithelial neoplasia in sexually active teenagers and young adults. Am J Obstet Gynecol 148: 726–729

Walker E M, Dodgson J, Duncan I D 1990 Is colposcopy of teenage women worthwhile? An eleven year review of teenage referrals in Dundee. J Gynaecol Surg 5: 391–394

Wilkinson C, Jones J M, McBride J 1990 Anxiety caused by abnormal result of a cervical smear test: a controlled trial. Br Med J 300: 440

Zaninetti P, Francheschi S, Baccolo M et al 1986 Characteristics of women under 20 with cervical intraepithelial neoplasia. Int J Epidemiol 15: 477–482

10

Recent advances in the treatment of advanced carcinoma of the cervix

R. D. Hunter   A. Brewster

Carcinoma of the cervix remains a major international health problem. In spite of a falling incidence in North America and Scandinavia, probably as a result of their cytology programmes, many European countries have not seen significant falls in incidence in the last two decades. In many developing countries, although accurate national statistics are not available, hospital figures suggest that carcinoma of the cervix is the commonest malignant disease in women. Prognosis is significantly related to the principal FIGO stages (0–IV) but even among the early stages prognosis can be poor in some subgroups (Pfeiffer et al 1989). Radical surgery (extended hysterectomy with cuff of vagina or radical Wertheim's hysterectomy) remains the best approach to the majority of patients with stages 0 and I disease because this treatment is curative in the majority and gives important prognostic information in the rest. Some patients with apparently early node negative disease do badly with conventional approaches. We need to identify those features which might allow the selection of patients who would benefit from more aggressive multimodality treatment regimens from the outset. Radical radiotherapy is the standard approach to the majority of patients with the higher stages of the disease and is the technique against which all potential advances must be tested. For the purpose of this chapter, advanced carcinoma will be patients with stage I disease who are unlikely to be cured by radical surgery as well as patients with stages II–IV disease.

For many decades clinicians managing carcinoma of the cervix have planned the individual patient's treatment with the limited information derived from clinical examination under anaesthesia supplemented by an intravenous urogram (IVU) and, in some centres, lymphangiography. The advances include improved imaging of the primary tumour and nodal metastatic disease, better biological assessment of the tumour, improved understanding of the place of radiotherapy following radical surgery and the place of surgery following radical X-ray therapy for a local bulky disease. The combination of these factors rather than any individual one offers hope for a more rational, successful and safer approach to patients with advanced carcinoma of the cervix. The individualization of treatment based on the assessment of the individual and her tumour may avoid unnecessary therapy for those patients who exhibit better prognostic features while focusing the effort on those who require it.

IMAGING

With the introduction of computed tomography (CT) scanning and then trans-rectal and trans-vaginal ultrasound, hopes were raised of improved pretreatment assessment of patients with localized primary disease. These methods have been disappointing and magnetic resonance imaging (MRI) is the only advance which has gained acceptance as the first new useful adjunct to previously established imaging techniques.

Magnetic resonance imaging

The advantages of MRI scanning are soft tissue definition, a larger field of view and the potential benefit of multiplanar imaging. The disadvantage is that it is time consuming to perform and some patients who have a tendency to claustrophobia are unable to tolerate the procedure. Primary carcinoma of the cervix and its extension into vagina, parametria, bladder, rectum and muscle is demonstrated as a high signal intensity mass on T2-weighted sequences (Fig. 10.1). T1-weighted sequences are useful to demonstrate enlarged pelvic or para-aortic lymph nodes and renal obstruction.

The presence and extent of parametrial infiltration is a critical factor in deciding whether surgical intervention is appropriate. CT scanning has a disappointing accuracy of only 30–58% in evaluating parametrial extension, errors in interpretation arising from parauterine blood vessels, nerves, lymphatics or fibrous tissue that may produce soft tissue strands within the parametria. Comparative studies have shown that MRI scanning is more accurate than CT scanning and clinical examination in determining the extent of parametrial infiltration (Kim et al 1990). Hricak et al (1988) assessed the accuracy of MRI scanning in 57 patients who subsequently underwent surgical evaluation and found a predictive value of 94% for determining the absence of parametrial disease. Overall, CT scanning has been shown to correlate with surgical findings in 60–70% of cases, whereas MRI provides accurate staging information in 70–90% of cases. MRI scanning does sometimes have difficulty in differentiating tissue oedema from tumour invasion, which may lead to an overestimate of tumour size. Both techniques have a similar accuracy of between 70% and 80% in detecting enlarged lymph nodes, and MRI scanning offers no diagnostic advantage over CT scanning in detecting whether enlarged nodes are simply hyperplastic or whether small foci of tumour are present in normal-size nodes.

More recently it has been shown that the assessment of tumour volume and the presence of enlarged pelvic or para-aortic nodes, as demonstrated on 25 patients with pretreatment MRI scanning, were better prognostic indicators than tumour stage (Hawnaur et al 1992). Eighty per cent of these patients

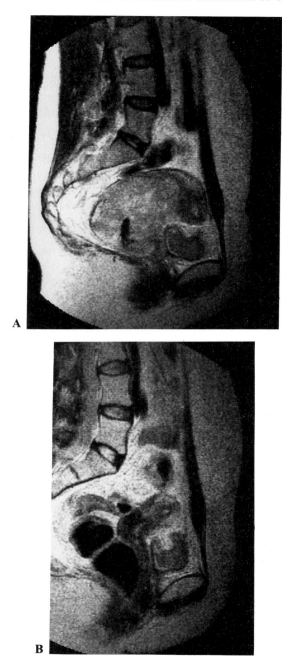

Fig. 10.1 T2-weighted sagittal MRI scan. **A** Patient with locally advanced carcinoma of the cervix. A very large soft tissue mass occupies the cervix and extends into the lower half of the uterus. The bladder is seen anteriorly and appears intact. **B** Post-treatment reconstitution of the cervix. The uterus is now of normal size.

with tumours greater than 40 cm³ developed local recurrence or metastases within 2 years of treatment. Follow-up scans performed at 1, 3, 6 and 12-month intervals showed that a less than 50% reduction in tumour bulk or a residual high signal intensity mass measuring greater than 10 cm³ on post-treatment MRI was associated with a poor outcome. This study further demonstrated that high signal intensity changes due to the effects of radiotherapy may be present for more than 2 years following treatment, making the diagnosis of recurrence difficult.

The ability of MRI scanning to define accurately the primary extent of disease and the benefits of multiplanar imaging suggests a role improving radiation planning. Russell et al (1992) used MRI scanning in 25 patients with stages IB–IVA carcinoma of the cervix to evaluate treatment fields that had been planned using conventional bony landmarks and clinical examination. They found that standard radiation portals would have resulted in a marginal miss (cancer outside treatment fields) in 6 patients and a potential miss (less than 1 cm margin) in a further 8 patients. In only 11 cases (44%) would the standard fields have adequately covered the primary tumour and its regional extension. Multiplanar images can also be obtained after placement of CT and MRI compatible intracavitary applicators allowing delineation of tumour extension in relation to the isodose distributions (Schoeppel et al 1992). These new approaches need an urgent assessment to determine the relationship between the information on the magnetic resonance image and that on a CT scan to ensure the benefits of both techniques for high-quality treatment planning.

HISTOLOGICAL AND BIOLOGICAL ASSESSMENT

Many attempts have been made over the years to relate prognosis in carcinoma of the cervix to histological parameters. Some patients, for example those with unusual small cell and carcinoid tumours, do very badly, but the majority of primary tumours are squamous cell, adeno and mixed adenosquamous types with different degrees of differentiation. No consensus has emerged that factors such as structure, differentiation, nuclear polymorphism, mitoses, extent and mode of invasion, lymphoplasmocytic cell response or vascular invasion can consistently be used between centres as reliable predictors or response to treatment and overall outcome. Perhaps the most successful attempt so far has been that of Haas & Friedl (1988), who analysed data from 583 patients with FIGO stages IB–IIB disease and using a multivariate approach identified four prognostic features which accurately predicted outcome in 80% of patients. The model was constructed using logistic regression analysis and was based on (1) the number of lymph nodes involved, (2) border zone and parametrial involvement, (3) exophytic tumour growth and (4) mitotic activity.

A very interesting feature of the last few years has been the investigation of possible biological parameters, and these are beginning to be examined prospectively in patients with carcinoma of the cervix. Those investigated recently include the following:

Tumour proliferation rate

Measurement of tumour growth fraction has previously been technically difficult, involving the incorporation of DNA precursors such as tritiated thymidine into tumour cells. Recently a monoclonal antibody, Ki67, which identifies nuclear antigen in human cells at all stages of the cell cycle except G_0, demonstrated good correlation with other methods of assessing tumour proliferation and correlated with a response to treatment in lymphomas. A prospective study of 28 patients with carcinoma of the cervix has shown no correlation between Ki67 staining and survival. In addition, no relationship was found with other prognostic parameters such as FIGO staging or node positivity (Cole et al 1992). This failure is disappointing but may in part reflect the small numbers studied to date, as the stain demonstrates considerable heterogeneity. Retrospective analysis is of limited value as the stain requires fresh material. A complex relationship probably exists between growth fraction and response to treatment, and a high growth fraction may not necessarily equate with poor prognosis.

DNA content

Rutgers et al (1986) found that in moderately and well-differentiated carcinomas of the cervix the non-diploid and non-tetraploid groups had an improved survival rate relative to the diploid and tetraploid tumours. This relationship was, however, not found in poorly differentiated tumours. Hanselaar et al (1990) looked at 37 cases of cervical intra-epithelial neoplasia (CIN) III and 32 of invasive carcinoma of the cervix and demonstrated no single specific DNA ploidy pattern which characterized the two lesions. However, cytophotometric techniques characterizing the nucleus using digitized images distinguished between CIN III and invasive carcinoma in 78% of cases. A retrospective study has failed to show a correlation between the degree of aneuploidy and prognosis (Davis et al 1989) and the relationship between DNA content in nuclei and prognosis in carcinoma of the cervix at present remains uncertain and requires further study.

c-myc oncogene

Amplification of the c-myc gene is observed in advanced carcinoma of the cervix and is associated with tumour progression. Riou et al (1990) studied 180 patients with carcinoma of the cervix and found a 6% over-expression in stages I and II compared with 37% in stages III and IV. Node-negative patients with normal expression of c-myc had a 93% survival rate compared with 51% where c-myc was over-expressed in a group of 93 patients followed for a mean of 30 months. An increase in the c-*myc* product, p62, has been shown to be associated with a decrease in disease-free survival rate and an increase in the rate of metastatic disease (Sowani et al 1989).

Epidermal growth factor

Pfeiffer et al (1989) measured epidermal growth factor and EGF receptor in 52 patients with carcinoma of the cervix compared with 40 biopsies from controls. Receptors with similar affinity were present in the normal cervix but cervical carcinoma demonstrated a higher binding capacity, suggesting an over-expression of the gene. Binding capacity within tumour tissue was heterogeneous but a higher EGF-like substance extracted from tumours positively correlated with lymph node metastases. Recurrence of disease and death was more common in patients with a high receptor capacity in that 43 of 45 patients with less than 100 fmol/mg protein showed no evidence of disease at 5 years compared with 2 out of 7 patients with a higher level of EGF receptor. The unequal numbers in each group, however, reduce its overall predictive value.

Squamous cell carcinoma antigen

Verlooy et al (1991) suggested that squamous cell carcinoma (SCC) antigen, measured in serum, directly and significantly correlated with stage of disease with a positivity rate of 50%. A study measuring SCC antigen levels in stage IB patients, however, failed to demonstrate any correlation between degree of elevation and extent of disease (Patsner et al 1989). All the patients were managed surgically and patients found to have para-aortic nodal metastases did not have raised antigen levels. No data were presented on recurrence or survival.

Human papillomavirus infection

With a strong association emerging between human papillomavirus (HPV) infection and primary carcinoma of the cervix, assessment of viral infection and the relationship to prognosis has been carried out. So far studies of the correlation between HPV infection and prognosis have failed to produce consistent results. Walker et al (1989) subjected 100 histologically confirmed SCCs of the cervix to DNA analysis. HPV DNA was present in 64 cases and limited follow-up (i.e. 20 months) suggested that HPV-18-positive tumours were more aggressive. In 69 stage IB tumours both a higher recurrence rate and statistically significant higher mortality were found when compared with those tumours which stained positively for HPV DNA-16 or did not stain at all. These changes were independent of histological type or grade. A retrospective multivariate analysis of HPV RNA in 212 patients found that the absence of detectable HPV RNA and advanced FIGO staging were independent risk factors (Higgins et al 1991). The authors found that the patients fell into two groups according to age, with a younger HPV RNA-positive group which did better than the older HPV RNA-negative group, who had a poorer prognosis.

Hypoxic fraction

A high initial hypoxic fraction associated with limited reoxygenation during treatment is thought to be one of the major factors influencing clinical response to radiotherapy (Adams 1990). Kolstad (1968) demonstrated a correlation between oxygen tension (pO_2) and tumour stage in carcinoma of the cervix, and controlled trials of hyperbaric oxygen in cervical carcinoma have shown significant benefit. Indirect evidence from histopathological analysis suggests that degree of vascularization may provide a significant prognostic factor (Siracky et al 1988), but more direct data of tumour oxygenation have been difficult to obtain with the existing technology. Recently oxygen histograms obtained using the Eppendorf histogram have demonstrated that mean pO_2 values in tumours are lower than those in normal tissues (Lartigau et al 1992). Hockel et al (1991) found that oxygenation patterns did not correlate with clinical stage or other parameters and suggest that tissue oxygenation may prove to be a useful independent prognostic indicator.

Prediction of radiotherapy response

Prediction of response to radiotherapy would be valuable in selecting the most appropriate combination of treatment strategies for patients with carcinoma of the cervix. The surviving fraction of carcinoma cells cultured from biopsies taken before radical radiotherapy and irradiated to 2 Gy in vitro (SF2) correlates with both local recurrence and survival assessed after a 2-year follow-up (West et al 1991). A significant difference in survival has been demonstrated in those patients with an SF2 greater than 0.55 compared with those with an SF2 less than this value. In addition, calculated probabilities of local recurrence were 57% with an SF2 greater than 0.55 compared with 5% for an SF2 less than 0.55. This project is being extended to involve more patients and to study normal tissue radiosensitivity in the individual patients, but at present intrinsic radiosensitivity is the most significant and exciting prognostic factor to have emerged from the biological investigation of human carcinoma of the cervix.

Further evaluation of the role of various biological prognostic factors including those outlined above is clearly required. In the future a scoring system may be devised which, by bringing together the most significant histological and biological factors, allows the clinician to select the most appropriate treatment combination for an individual patient. Undoubtedly many more biological prognostic factors will have to be assessed both individually and together before a clinically secure biological index emerges.

TREATMENT

Radiotherapy after radical surgery

The pathological assessment of the radical hysterectomy specimen using a modern approach gives a comprehensive picture of the biological behaviour of the individual's disease. In addition to the histological type and grading of the primary tumour and its volume, the margin of excision in relation to the vagina and parametrium should be available. Information about vascular space invasion both within veins and lymphatics is also helpful. The assessment of nodal disease should include the number, site and size of the nodes received as well as the number and nature of any malignant infiltration and extranodal spread.

In patients free from evidence of para-aortic nodal disease, the post-hysterectomy patients can be split into different prognostic groupings depending on the presence or absence of poor histological prognostic features in the primary tumour and/or involved pelvic lymph nodes.

A retrospective analysis of 141 surgically treated patients with stages I and IIA disease (Buxton et al 1990) identified depth of invasion, substage, lymph node involvement, lymphatic and blood vessel invasion and tumour differentiation as significant prognostic variables. After stratification for depth of invasion, (1) substage, (2) lymphatic and blood vessel invasion and (3) tumour differentiation emerged as independent prognostic variables. The authors have gone on to develop classification models which in a further group of patients treated by surgery and radiation therapy have identified a subgroup of approximately one-third of the overall group in whom they predicted a high probability of relapse. At the time of publication this had occurred in 60% of the poor-risk group within 18 months of treatment. This approach needs further assessment by other centres, but if it is sustained identification of 'early' stage patients who required postoperative adjuvant therapy including radiotherapy and/or chemotherapy would be much easier and their treatment more consistent.

A recent retrospective analysis of 249 patients with stage IB disease treated by Wertheim's hysterectomy in a major US cancer centre (Larson et al 1988) adds the information that 89% of recurrences occur in the first 2 years and that approximately half of the patients with recurrence confined to the pelvis or vulva can be salvaged by subsequent radiation therapy. Further work needs to be done to separate prospectively patients with recurrent disease to allow the radio-curable patients to avoid unnecessary systemic treatment.

Surgery after radical radiotherapy

A special group which has helped to create much confusion over the last two decades has been those patients with stage I bulky endocervical carcinoma in whom some authors have suggested that 'a subfascial hysterectomy' should be performed after radical radiotherapy. Taking this to mean primary tumours greater than 6 cm in diameter, Thomas et al (1992) could find no correlation between substage and pelvic control or survival rate. On the other hand, 'volume' as defined by greater or less than 8 cm in diameter emerged as a very significant and important prognostic factor. Multivariate analysis of the results failed to draw any firm conclusion about the value of adjuvant surgery because the study was not randomized, but the authors noted a shift in their centre away from routine post-radiotherapy hysterectomy and felt that the place of planned surgery after radiotherapy was not supported by their data.

In selecting patients for combined approach, improved biological assessment of the radiosensitivity of the primary tumour and of the individual and prospective monitoring of the response of the tumour to therapy using the biological and imaging techniques of the type described above may prove to be a more acceptable approach to this problem.

Another important observation that needs further assessment in this important subgroup is that it has been suggested (Whitaker et al 1990) that good cytological follow-up of the primary tumour in the post-radiotherapy period may help to identify the patient with localized disease who is failing to resolve satisfactorily with a sensitivity of 85% and a specificity of 99.5%. There has for many years been a reluctance to use this approach because after radical radiotherapy cytological assessment needs considerable experience to distinguish significant malignant cell changes from the normal radiotherapy-induced cellular changes. This approach has been tried intermittently over the past few decades but further assessment is needed using modern cytological techniques since smears are easily obtained at follow-up. Unfortunately cytological follow-up has the potential for increased anxiety in the patient shedding malignant-looking cells although actually resolving satisfactorily. This can present difficulties for the physician responsible.

Para-aortic irradiation

A further special subgroup comprises patients with para-aortic lymph node invasion at the time of initial treatment. They have been very difficult to identify in the past without surgical dissection. This type of spread is recognized to be correlated with bulky primary tumours and the higher stages and as a result some groups have advocated prophylactic irradiation in subgroups at risk. Unfortunately, experience in the EORTC and the RTOG 7920 trial (Rotman et al 1990) with radical radiotherapy has shown that the routine extension of the radiation fields to include the para-aortic region in patients with bulky advanced primary disease does not improve survival and is associated with increased morbidity. A more positive finding comes from a recent analysis of the impact of extended field radiotherapy after para-aortic lymph node dissection in patients with histologically proven para-aortic disease (Lovecchio et al 1989). This showed an encouraging 50% 5-year actuarial survival without any major radiotherapy complication. In this study, 75% of patients who did relapse did so outside the irradiated volume, emphasizing the need to consider systemic therapy if results are to be further improved in this group of patients. Routine para-aortic lymph node dissection is likely to increase overall morbidity, and techniques aimed at developing specificity with minimally invasive imaging approaches offer promise for the selection of subgroups for trials of new forms of systemic therapy.

Radical radiotherapy in advanced disease

In locally advanced carcinoma of the cervix treated with standard radical radiotherapy techniques, a number of papers over the last few years have pointed to the inadequacy of the present substaging of both stage II and stage III. These papers include the recently reported multicentre American Patterns of Care Study (PCS) (Lanciano et al 1991). This concludes that unilateral parametrial invasion in stage IIB and unilateral fixation in stage IIIB are significant positive prognostic features with respect to survival after radical radiotherapy treatment. The study also demonstrated that FIGO substaging did not significantly predict survival and it supports the growing evidence for a reappraisal and refinement of the staging system. Tumour volume rather than tissue involvement is likely to become increasingly important as different adjuvant approaches are considered in this disease. The confident identification and separation of good prognostic groups of patients from poor prognostic groups within each FIGO stage would allow better patient selection and ensure an absence of preventable bias between groups in future adjuvant studies.

Towards improving radical radiotherapy

Over the years many attempts have been made to improve the results in locally advanced stage II and III disease by combining standard radiotherapy techniques with modalities like hyperbaric oxygen, hypoxic cell sensitizers and high-energy neutrons. Hyperbaric oxygen proved efficacious but impractical; hypoxic sensitizers have so far proved to be too toxic for conventional use; and neutrons are no more successful than photons but are associated with a higher morbidity and mortality. Two more modern approaches are under continuing scrutiny by different groups. The most widespread approach involves trials of neo-adjuvant chemotherapy. It is recognized that patients given platinum-based combination chemotherapy prior to radical radiotherapy can show relatively high combined complete and partial responses and that the responders are more likely to survive following their radiotherapy (Symonds et al 1989). This appears so far to be possible without an increase in acute or late morbidity, and as a consequence a number of UK-based groups coordinated by the United Kingdom Coordinating Committee for

Cancer Research (UKCCCR) gynaecological subgroup are pursuing this approach with randomized trials. It seems likely that none of them individually will be definitive but this approach will lend itself eventually to an international metanalysis along the lines of those in breast and ovarian carcinoma which have been so helpful in sorting out the place of early adjuvant treatment.

The previously mentioned PCS also confirmed a long-held radiotherapy prejudice that the best results in advanced carcinoma of the cervix are achieved by combining external beam radiotherapy with intracavitary treatment. The relative value of intracavitary therapy and its type — low dose rate or high dose rate — are the subject of vigorous debate by different protagonists but there is at present no evidence that there is a definite therapeutic advantage with one particular approach, and there is suspicion that optimum schedules with different balances of external and internal treatment and different types of afterloading will produce equivalent results. The choice presented to the radiotherapists by the development of satisfactory remote afterloading equipment of both low and high rate type seems likely to remain to be biased by personal experience, patient workload, the availability of anaesthesia, beds and nursing support. The high dose rate techniques are labour intensive for medical and scientific staff, while the burden of low dose rate techniques falls on the wards and nursing staff.

Another approach to advanced carcinoma of the cervix has developed from the renaissance of brachytherapy techniques allowed by the introduction of computer-controlled afterloading machines and new artificial radionuclides. A very old, parametrial interstitial technique developed in the heyday of radium therapy has been modified to a fixed-geometry pelvic template which allows the placement through the perineum of multiple interstitial hollow needles which then act as the carriers for caesium-137 or irridium-192 sources. Martinez et al (1985) have refined earlier techniques and claim that in selected locally advanced disease patients' improved survival rates and local control can be achieved without a dramatic increase in morbidity. The success of the technique lies in its ability to extend active treatment more laterally than is possible with the classical uterine and vaginal intracavitary brachytherapy applicators and their limited pear-shaped dose distribution. The technique involves the use of special skills which are not yet widely available, and the opportunity to test this approach against the optimal alternative radiotherapy and combined radiotherapy and chemotherapy regimes would need a multicentre study.

CHEMOTHERAPY

The introduction of cisplatin into oncology, better non-invasive imaging techniques for the pelvis, and an increasing number of younger patients with advanced and recurrent carcinoma of the cervix during the 1980s, have led to an extensive reassessment of the value of chemotherapy in this disease. Using different techniques for assessment of response, many groups have published results detailing their experience with single-agent and combination chemotherapy with widely different claims about responsiveness. Reviewing the area, Albert & Mason-Liddil (1989) concluded that although objective responses of up to 65% and complete response rates of up to 36% have been recorded, there is still little evidence to suggest that the effect of cisplatin is enhanced by the use of any other drugs, and there is a clear understanding that chemotherapy of any type is rarely followed by good maintained remission.

Among other agents, ifosfamide, methotrexate, 5-fluorouracil and mitomycin C are regularly used in combination with cisplatin in the treatment of recurrent disease, without any one emerging as being any better than any other.

As in most solid tumour situations experience has first been gained by a single agent on recurrent disease. This inevitably means patients with advanced or recurrent carcinoma of the cervix who have previously had radiotherapy and in whom there is often a degree of obstructive uropathy. Given the difficulties involved, it is not surprising that no consensus view has emerged. Chemotherapy for recurrent disease still has a role in the younger symptomatic patient and in particular those with pulmonary metastases, but if early response is not achieved chemotherapy should be discontinued.

The relatively good partial responses seen in patients with recurrent disease given chemotherapy have encouraged more groups to consider the use of chemotherapy as part of the initial management scheme. This has previously been mentioned in relation to radiotherapy, but a logical extension is to use it prior to or following radical surgery in patients with locally advanced disease or poor prognostic tumours. Combined pretreatment responses of 80% (Leminen et al 1992) in response to presurgical systemic combination chemotherapy is very encouraging and needs careful prospective study by collaborative groups. Some of these are ongoing in the form of synchronous and neo-adjuvant therapy and the results are not going to be available for about 5 years.

In view of the lack of consensus emerging from studies of the newer agents it is pertinent that we are reminded by Stehman et al (1992) about hydroxyurea, which remains the most successful radiosensitizing drug in carcinoma of the cervix and has been shown to produce improved survival in patients treated with a combination of approaches in several randomized trials.

CONCLUSION

Advanced carcinoma of the cervix remains a major clinical challenge. Some of the developments discussed above and extensions of them will undoubtedly lead to management improvements in the future. Locally bulky tumours are always going to be difficult to clear. The numbers of patients entered into clinical trials in this area remain very low relative to the numbers of patients with the disease, and the rate of improvement is going to be directly related to the willingness of clinicians to participate in collective studies in the future.

KEY POINTS FOR CLINICAL PRACTICE

1. Magnetic resonance scanning offers vastly improved imaging in the pretreatment assessment of patients with primary advanced carcinoma of the cervix.

2. Subfascial hysterectomy is not indicated as a routine procedure after primary radical radiotherapy of locally bulky tumour.

3. Para-aortic irradiation should be reserved for patients with known para-aortic involvement.

4. Radical radiotherapy is likely to improve with better patient individualization in treatment planning based on improved imaging and knowledge of biological features of the tumour.

REFERENCES

Adams G E 1990 The clinical relevance of tumour hypoxia. Eur J Cancer 26: 420–421
Albert D S, Mason-Liddil N 1989 The role of cisplatin in the management of advanced squamous cell cancer of the cervix. Semin Oncol 16 (4 suppl 6): 66–78
Buxton E J, Saunders N, Blackledge G et al 1990 The potential for adjuvant therapy in early stage cervical cancer. Cancer Chemother Pharmacol 26: 17–21
Cole D J, Brown D C, Crossley E et al 1992 Carcinoma of the cervix uteri: an assessment of the relationship of tumour proliferation to prognosis. Br J Cancer 65: 783–785
Davis J R, Aristizabal S, Way D L et al 1989 DNA ploidy, grade and stage in prognosis of uterine cervical cancer. Gynaecol Oncol 32: 4–7
Haas J, Friedl H 1988 Prognostic factors in cervical carcinoma: a multivariate approach. In: Baillière's Clinical obstetrics and gynaecology Vol. 2(4). Baillière Tindall, London, pp 829–837
Hanselaar A G J M, Vooijs G P, Pahlplatz M M M 1990 DNA ploidy and cytophotometric analysis of cervical intraepithelial neoplasia grade III and invasive squamous cell carcinoma. Cytometry II: 624–629
Hawnaur J M, Johnson R J, Hunter R D et al 1992 The value of magnetic resonance imaging in assessment of carcinoma of the cervix and its response to radiotherapy. Clin Oncol 4: 11–17
Higgins G D, Davy M, Roder D et al 1991 Increased age and mortality associated with cervical carcinoma negative for human papillomavirus RNA. Lancet 388: 910–913
Hricak H, Lacey C G, Sandles L G et al 1988 Invasive cervical carcinoma: comparison of MR imaging and surgical findings. Radiology 166: 623–631
Hockel M, Schlenger K, Knoop C, Vaupel P 1991 Oxygenation of carcinomas of the uterine cervix: evaluation by computerized oxygen tension measurements. Cancer Res 51: 6098–6102
Kim S H, Choi B I, Lee H P et al 1990 Uterine cervical carcinoma: comparison of CT and MR findings. Radiology 175: 45–51
Kolstad P 1968 Intercapillary distance, oxygen tension and local recurrence in cervix cancer. Scand J Clin Lab Invest 106: 145–157
Lanciano R, Won M, Coia L, Hanks G 1991 Pretreatment and treatment factors associated with improved outcome in squamous cell carcinoma of the uterine cervix. Int J Radiat Oncol Biol Phys 20: 667–676
Larson D, Ropeland L, Stringer C et al 1988 Recurrent cervical cancer after radical hysterectomy. Gynaecol Oncol 30: 381–387
Lartigau E, Vitu E, Haie-Meder C et al 1992 Feasibility of measuring oxygen tension in

uterine cervix carcinoma. Eur J Cancer 28A: 1354–1357

Leminen A, Alfton H, Stenham U, Lentovirta P 1992 Chemotherapy as initial treatment for cervical cancer. Acta Obstet Gynaecol Scand 71: 293–297

Lovecchio J, Arerette H E, Donato D, Bell J 1989 5 year survival of patients with peri-aortic nodal metastases in clinical stage IB and IIA cervical carcinoma. Gynaecol Oncol 34: 43–45

Martinez A, Edmundson G K, Cox R S et al 1985 Combination of external beam irradiation and multiple-site perineal applicator (MUPIT) for treatment of locally advanced or recurrent prostatic, anorectal and gynaecological malignancies. Int J Radiat Oncol Biol Phys 11: 391–398

Patsner B, Orr J W, Allmen T 1989 Does pre-operative serum squamous cell carcinoma antigen level predict occult extracervical disease in patients with stage Ib invasive squamous cell carcinoma of the cervix? Obstet Gynaecol 74: 786–788

Pfeiffer D, Stellwag B, Pfeiffer A et al 1989 Clinical implications of the epidermal growth factor receptor in the squamous cell carcinoma of the uterine cervix. Gynaecol Oncol 33: 146–150

Riou G F, Bourhis J, Le M G 1990 The c-myc proto-oncogene in invasive carcinomas of the uterine cervix: clinical relevance of over expression in early stages of the cancer. Anticancer Res 10: 1225–1232

Rotman M, Choi K, Guse C et al 1990 Prophylactic irradiation of the para-aortic lymph node chain in stage IIB and bulky stage IB carcinoma of the cervix. Int J Radiat Oncol Biol Phys 19: 415–521

Russell A H, Walter J P, Anderson M W, Zukowski C L 1992 Sagittal magnetic resonance imaging in the design of lateral radiation treatment portals for patients with locally advanced squamous cancer of the cervix. Int J Radiat Oncol Biol Phys 23: 449–455

Rutgers D H, vander Linden P, van Peperzeel H A 1986 DNA flow cytometry of squamous cell carcinomas from the human uterine cervix: the identification of prognostically different subgroups. Radiother Oncol 7: 249–258

Schoeppel S L, Ellis J H, LaVigne M L et al 1992 Magnetic resonance imaging during intracavitary gynaecological brachytherapy. Int J Radiat Oncol Biol Phys 23:169–74

Siracky J, Siracka E, Kovac R, Revesz L 1988 Prognostic significance of vascular density and a malignancy grading in radiation treated uterine cervix carcinoma. Neoplasma 35: 289–296

Sowani A, Ong G, Dische S et al 1989 c-myc oncogene expression and clinical outcome in carcinoma of the cervix. Mol Cell Probes 3: 117–123

Stehman F B 1992 Experience with hydroxyurea as a radiosensitizer in carcinoma of the cervix. Semin Oncol 19 (3 suppl 9): 48–52

Symonds R P, Burnett R A, Habeshaw T 1989 The prognostic value of a response to chemotherapy given before radiotherapy in advanced cancer of the cervix. Br J Cancer 59: 473–475

Thomas W, Eifel P, Smith T et al 1992 Bulky endocervical carcinoma: a 23 year experience. Int J Radiat Oncol Biol Phys 23: 491–499

Verlooy H, Devos P, Janssens J et al 1991 Clinical significance of squamous cell carcinoma antigen in cancer of the human uterine cervix: comparison with CEA and Ca-125. Gynaecol Obstet Invest 32: 55–58

Walker J, Bloss J D, Liao S Y et al 1989 Human papillomavirus genotype as a prognostic indicator in carcinoma of the uterine cervix. Obstet Gynaecol 74: 781–785

West C M L, Davidson S E, Hendry J H, Hunter R D 1991 Predication of cervical carcinoma response to radiotherapy. Lancet 338: 818

Whitaker S, Blake P, Trott P 1990 The value of cervical cytology in detecting recurrent squamous carcinoma of the cervix post radiotherapy. Clin Oncol 2: 254–259

11

Update on chemotherapy for advanced ovarian cancer

L. A. Stewart   D. Guthrie

Ovarian cancer is the seventh most common cancer of women. Worldwide, some 140 000 new cases are diagnosed each year and the disease is responsible for the greatest number of deaths from gynaecological malignancy in Europe and North America (Parkin et al 1980).

Unlike cancers of the corpus and cervix uteri, ovarian cancers give few early warnings. The disease is largely asymptomatic in its early stages and around 70% of patients present with advanced intra-abdominal disease, by which time prognosis is usually very poor. The symptom most commonly reported at presentation is abdominal distension, but patients may also complain of a variety of other abdominal symptoms. Postmenopausal or other abnormal vaginal bleeding is reported less frequently.

For early-stage disease [International Federation of Gynaecology and Obstetrics (FIGO) I–IIa], 5-year survival rates are around 50–70%, whereas with advanced tumours the corresponding survival rates fall to 5–10%. It has been suggested that the disappointingly low survival in advanced disease (FIGO III and IV) could be potentially improved by early detection. However, there is currently no evidence that screening, either with CA125 or by transvaginal ultrasonography, improves survival (Granai 1992). At present, hope for progress rests mainly on improving treatments.

Maximum cytoreductive surgery is considered the most effective first-line therapy for all tumour stages. Indeed, for stage I disease, surgery is often the only recommended treatment and usually consists of total abdominal hysterectomy and bilateral salpingo-oophorectomy and omentectomy. For patients with advanced disease, tumour debulking is usually followed by some form of chemotherapy.

Ovarian cancer was one of the first solid malignant tumours to be treated with chemotherapy, and the single alkylating agents that were used over 30 years ago were considered optimal treatment for advanced disease until the mid-1970s. Since then, therapeutic practice has undergone a series of changes as summarized in Fig. 11.1. Following the publication of a small trial which reported that HexaCAF (hexamethylmelamine, methotrexate, cyclophosphamide and fluorouracil) achieved higher response rates than melphalan alone (Young et al 1978), the use of drug combinations became

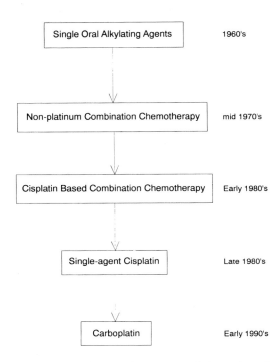

Fig. 11.1   Trends in the chemotherapeutic treatment of advanced ovarian cancer.

widespread. Around the same time cisplatin, which had shown efficacy in phase II trials (Wiltshaw & Kroner 1976), became available and was quickly incorporated into multidrug regimens. Later, when the effectiveness of doxorubicin was questioned and a number of randomized trials failed to show significant differences between cisplatin given as a single agent and cisplatin-based combination chemotherapy, many centres adopted cisplatin alone as routine first-line treatment. Recently, the use of carboplatin both as a single agent and in combination with other drugs has become common.

These changes in disease management have taken place on the basis of very little good evidence. Although there have been many randomized studies comparing different chemotherapy regimens, these have not had sufficient numbers of patients to show clear benefit of one form of chemotherapy over another. For example, 700 patients would be required to detect a 10% absolute improvement in 2-year survival from 20% to 30% with reliability (5% test size 90% power) (MRC GCWP 1990). The largest published two-arm trial (Brodovsky et al 1984) reported on 374 patients. It therefore remains unclear what constitutes optimum chemotherapy for advanced ovarian cancer, and standard treatment strategies vary both nationally and internationally.

An exhaustive meta-analysis based on individual patient data from trials investigating the role of chemotherapy in advanced ovarian cancer has recently been published (AOCTG 1991). This project, which analysed information from 45 randomized clinical trials, over 8000 patients and almost 6500 deaths, represents the most comprehensive review of chemotherapy ever undertaken in this disease. This chapter reviews some of the results and discusses the implications of this study as well as considering other recent developments in the treatment of advanced ovarian cancer.

THE ADVANCED OVARIAN CANCER OVERVIEW (META-ANALYSIS)

The advanced ovarian cancer overview (AOCO) was carried out on behalf of the international Advanced Ovarian Cancer Trialists Group (AOCTG) to consider the role of platinum and combination chemotherapy in advanced disease. The AOCO aimed to synthesize and evaluate the evidence from previous clinical research, both to determine the 'best' of currently available types of treatment and to establish reliable foundations for future research. Formal meta-analyses were carried out for each of the five separate comparisons considered in the overview (Table 11.1). The *results* of individual trials were combined within each comparison using formal methodology to compute the relative risk associated with each of the treatments in question. This gives the relative risk of death associated with the two types of treatment. When comparing 'control' against 'treatment', a relative risk of less than 1.0 favours the treatment arm, a value of 1.0 indicates no difference between the two arms, whilst a value of greater than 1.0 favours the control arm. For example, a relative risk of 0.8 represents a 20% decrease in the risk of death when using the treatment arm.

The wide variety of treatments tested in ovarian cancer trials did not allow analysis of specific regimens but led to trials being grouped according to the type of drug that they compared. Nevertheless the results of the overview offer the most reliable estimates of the efficacy of various types of chemotherapy currently available. The most important of the results which are presented in Table 11.1 are discussed below.

Results of the AOCO (meta-analysis)

Non-platinum regimens versus platinum-based combination chemotherapy

The analysis of 1329 patients from 11 randomized trials comparing a single

Table 11.1 Summary of the results of the advanced ovarian cancer overview

Comparison	Available trials	Unavailable trials	Patients	Deaths	Log rank χ^2	p-value (1 d.f.)	Relative risk	95% confidence interval
(a) Single non-platinum agent versus non-platinum combination	16	6	3146	2817	0.65	0.42	0.98	0.91–1.05
(b) Single non-platinum agent versus platinum combination	11	2	1329	1136	1.09	0.30	0.93	0.83–1.05
(c) Non-platinum regimen versus same regimen plus platinum	8	0	1408	1134	2.8	0.10	0.91	0.81–1.02
(d) Single-agent platinum versus platinum-based combination	6	0	925	712	2.53	0.11	0.89	0.76–1.04
(e) As (d) but excluding high-dose/low-dose study	5	0	838	634	4.82	0.03	0.85	0.72–1.00
(f) Cisplatin versus carboplatin	11	0	2061	1771	0.91	0.34	1.05	0.94–1.18

non-platinum drug against a platinum-based combination showed no significant difference between the two treatments (Table 11.1b). The survival curves (Fig. 11.2) show an initial separation in favour of combination chemotherapy but converge by year 6. The relative risk of 0.93 suggests a 7% reduction in risk in favour of platinum-based treatment, although the observed trend is not significant in a formal statistical sense.

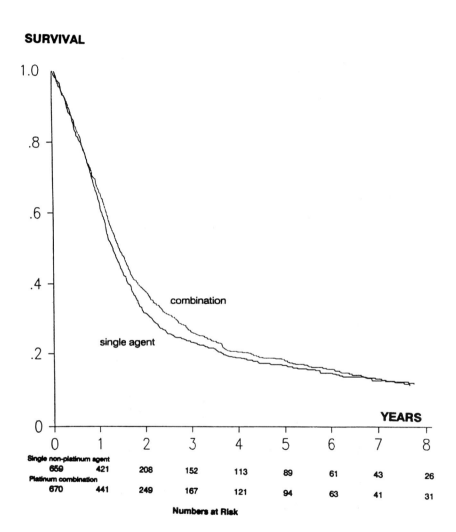

Fig. 11.2   Survival curves comparing a single non-platinum drug with a platinum-based combination. Reproduced with permission from the British Medical Association and Advanced Ovarian Cancer Trialists Group (1991).

This particular comparison might have been expected to show the largest treatment effect as it compared what is often regarded as the least intensive form of treatment with the most intensive, but the trend favouring combination chemotherapy was not statistically significant. However, only one trial (Crowther et al, unpublished) precluded the use of platinum-based therapy on relapse for those patients initially allocated single non-platinum drugs. Thus, in effect the comparison may be better summarized as immediate versus deferred platinum therapy.

A similar analysis of 1408 patients from eight trials comparing a platinum-based combination with the same regimen minus the platinum-based drug showed a comparable survival pattern, also with a non-significant trend in favour of the platinum-based combinations (Table 11.1c). The doses of cisplatin used in these trials were similar and additional drugs were common to both arms of each trial, making this a more clear-cut comparison. There were, however, similar problems associated with patients receiving platinum-based treatment on relapse.

Single-agent platinum versus platinum-based combination chemotherapy

The analysis of data from 925 patients from six randomized trials comparing single-agent platinum with a platinum combination gave a different survival pattern. The survival curves based on a median follow-up of 6.5 years (Fig. 11.3) suggest a difference in favour of the combination chemotherapy after 2 years that is maintained until about year 8, although this trend is also non-significant (Table 11.1d). The relative risk of 0.89 suggests an 11% reduction in the risk of death associated with the multiple drug regimens. Further, when one trial (Wiltshaw et al 1986) which compared high-dose cisplatin alone with low-dose cisplatin in combination (with other cytotoxic drugs) was excluded from the analysis, this trend in favour of platinum combinations was marginally significant (Table 11.1e).

A possible explanation for the difference in survival pattern between this comparison and those described previously might be that in this case both treatment groups received some form of immediate platinum-based therapy. Thus the comparison did not suffer from the problem of 'control' patients receiving platinum on relapse. It should be noted, however, that most trials used platinum as a single agent at a dose lower than is currently recommended and it is therefore unclear whether the observed trend in favour of combination therapy was due to the effect of additional drugs per se or to the increased total drug dose of the combination chemotherapy.

Cisplatin versus carboplatin

An analysis based on 2061 patients from 11 randomized trials comparing carboplatin against cisplatin both on their own and in combination with other drugs showed there to be no difference in survival between the two analogues

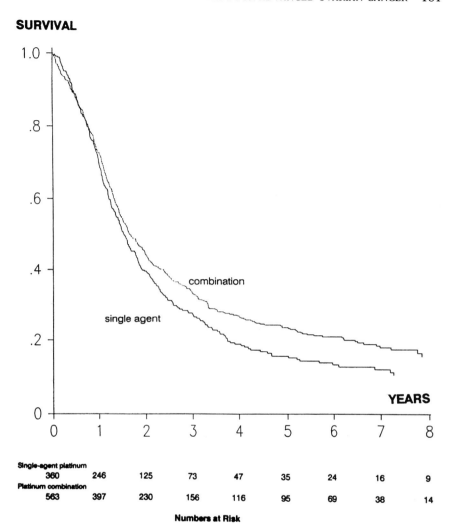

Fig. 11.3 Survival curves comparing single-agent platinum with platinum based combination. Reproduced with permission from the British Medical Association and Advanced Ovarian Cancer Trialists Group (1991).

(Table 11.1f, Fig 11.4). However, the median follow-up on these trials was only 3 years, reflecting their relatively recent nature, and a future updated analysis is planned. It should also be noted that in these trials carboplatin dose was based on surface area rather than renal clearance as is currently recommended. Nevertheless the results of this comparison offer no good evidence at this time that cisplatin is either superior or inferior to carboplatin in terms of survival.

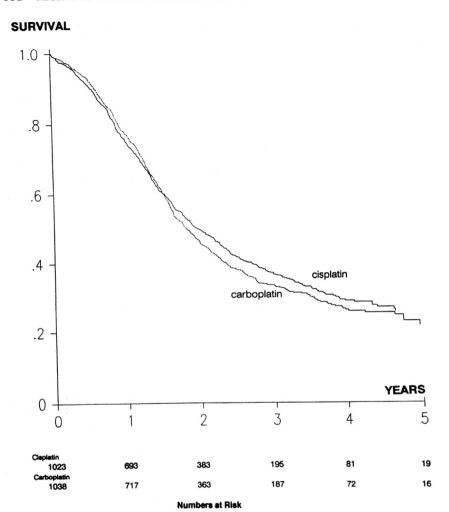

Fig. 11.4   Survival curves comparing cisplatin and carboplatin. Reproduced with permission from the British Medical Association and Advanced Ovarian Cancer Trialists Group (1991).

Interpretation of the results of the AOCO (meta-analysis)

In contrast to the curative potential of chemotherapy in some cancers, such as testicular teratoma, it is clear that chemotherapy has not yet achieved substantial benefits in advanced ovarian cancer. However, moderate improvements may have been gained, which although not dramatic could be extremely important in public health terms in view of the relatively high incidence of the disease. For example, even a moderate improvement in survival of around 5% could prolong the lives of thousands of women throughout the world each year. The AOCO was planned to try to detect such moderate differences with reliability. However, all but one of the confidence intervals presented in Table 11.1 span a relative risk value of 1.0, indicating that the results could be consistent with a beneficial, equivalent, or detrimental treatment effect. For example the 95% confidence interval for the relative risk calculated for trials comparing single-agent platinum with platinum combinations 0.81–1.02, which is consistent with a 9% benefit in the overall risk of death associated with combination chemotherapy and also with a 2% detrimental effect. From this it is clear that even the combination of many trials does not provide sufficient numbers of patients to make *firm* statements about the results. Although the results suggest possible benefit from immediate platinum-based combination chemotherapy no absolutely conclusive evidence emerged.

Although these results may on first inspection appear rather disheartening, there are important lessons to be learned from the overview which has raised three important hypotheses:

1. Platinum combinations are generally better than non-platinum regimens as first-line therapy.
2. Platinum combinations are generally better than single-agent platinum when platinum is given at the same dose.
3. Cisplatin and carboplatin are equally effective.

The role of doxorubicin (Adriamycin)

The proposition that adding other drugs to cisplatin may improve survival is supported by the results of another independent meta-analysis, the CAP/CP overview (OCM-AP 1991). This project investigated the role of doxorubicin in advanced ovarian cancer and found that the CAP (cyclophosphamide, doxorubicin, cisplatin) regimen was significantly more effective in terms of survival than CP, with an estimated 15% reduction in the odds of death associated with CAP.

Combination chemotherapy

The proposed effectiveness of combination chemotherapy may be attributed to either, or both, of two possible mechanisms. First, combinations can include drugs which have different modes of action and which therefore could have synergistic effects. Second, the total combined dose of drugs, irrespective of drug type, is greater so that the tumour cells are exposed to a higher concentration of cytotoxic agents. Patients could therefore have derived a benefit either from receiving a higher total dose of cytotoxics (which could also be potentially achieved by giving a high dose of a single agent), or from a synergism between drugs, or possibly from a combination of the two. Consideration of the results of the AOCO and the CAP/CP overview therefore leads to the important question: when given at maximum tolerated dose, is platinum-based combination chemotherapy or single-agent cisplatin/carboplatin the 'best' of current standard treatments?

The icon-2 trial

A large international trial, icon-2 (International Collaborative Ovarian Neoplasm — Study 2), has been undertaken to try to answer the above question. Carboplatin is being used as the single-agent platinum compound since it is less emetogenic and less nephrotoxic, although more myelosuppressive than cisplatin and has the added advantage of out-patient treatment. Based on the results of both the AOCO and the CAP/CP overview, CAP is being used as the combination chemotherapy. Although some of the severe side-effects of CAP can be controlled by the use of anti-emetic agents such as ondansetron, it is certainly more toxic than carboplatin. However, only with a reliable estimate of any survival improvement can a cost–benefit assessment of treatments including survival, toxicity, quality of life and cost be performed. Studies of patients' attitudes have shown that they are willing to accept more aggressive therapies in return for very modest survival benefits (Slevin et al 1990). A conventionally 'null' result would also be important as the lower toxicity of single-agent carboplatin would, in this case, make it likely to be the treatment of choice.

In icon-2, carboplatin is given at 'full' dosage with adjustment for glomerular filtration rate (Calvert et al 1989). The CAP regimen consists of cyclophosphamide 500 mg/m^2 and doxorubicin 50 mg/m^2, both given as intravenous bolus injections, and 50 mg/m^2 of cisplatin infused over 30 minutes or longer with adequate hydration before, during and after treatment. In both cases, six cycles of chemotherapy are given at 3-week intervals. These dose schedules have been chosen in order that drugs should be given in 'full' dose as quickly as possible.

Participation in the trial has been made as simple as possible. Any patient with histologically confirmed epithelial ovarian carcinoma whom the clinician is certain requires some form of immediate chemotherapy is eligible. Randomization requires only a simple telephone call to the trial centre and form filling is minimal. The trial plans to recruit 2000 patients worldwide. To accrue such a large number of patients a number of such trials are being carried out in parallel. Each is independently managed but all are coordinated on an international basis and the results of each will be pooled in the final analysis in a manner analogous to a multicentre trial.

If successful the trial will help delineate 'best current practice' (Whitehouse 1989) and also provide the standard treatment for future studies.

OTHER DEVELOPMENTS

Dose intensity

Recently there has been considerable interest in the idea of delivering as much drug as possible to the tumour as quickly as possible, and there has been much speculation about the role of both dose and dose intensity of chemotherapy in treating ovarian tumours. Interest in dose intensity, which can be defined as the amount of drug delivered per week, irrespective of scheduling, stems from laboratory studies and the publication of a retrospective analysis. In this analysis, which claimed that dose intensity was a determinant of treatment outcome in ovarian cancer patients (Levin & Hryniuk 1987), dose intensity was calculated relative to a chosen standard of the CHAP (cyclophosphamide, hexamethylmelamine, doxorubicin and cisplatin) regimen. The average relative dose intensity, especially of cisplatin, was found to be associated with both clinical response and median survival time. However, there are many difficulties with the methodology used, not least of which was the poor quality of available data and the subsequent major assumptions required in the analysis. Nevertheless, the results stimulated much interest in the idea of dose intensity, especially with regard to platinum-based therapy.

Two randomized trials comparing high-dose against low-dose cisplatin-based treatment have recently been published. The first of these (Kaye et al 1992) compared 50 mg/m^2 (low-dose) with 100 mg/m^2 (high-dose) cisplatin, both given with 750 mg/m^2 cyclophosphamide at 3-weekly intervals for a maximum of six courses. This trial of 165 patients found that progression-free survival and overall survival were significantly improved for those patients receiving the high-dose regimen, but at the expense of significantly worse side-effects. The second study of 485 patients (McGuire et al 1992) compared 50 mg/m^2 cisplatin plus 500 mg/m^2 cyclophosphamide for eight cycles with 100 mg/m^2 cisplatin plus 1000 mg/m^2 cyclophosphamide for only four cycles. This study found no difference in overall response of median survival between the two treatments, although toxicity was more severe in the high-dose arm. In the Kaye trial, both the dose intensity and total dose varied between treatment arms and it is therefore not clear whether the observed difference in survival was due to the increased total cumulative drug dose or to the increased dose intensity. In the McGuire trial the total dose remained constant whilst the dose intensity doubled. Taking the results of these trials together suggests that dose intensity may be less important than total drug dose, and currently there is insufficient evidence to judge whether dose intensity is clinically important. Clearly, further research into drug dose and scheduling is warranted. However, it is clear from the experience of these trials that the burden of toxicity is unacceptable with such high dose schedules and that these should not at present be adopted into routine clinical practice. Such treatments should only be considered as options within a randomized clinical trial.

High-dose carboplatin may offer a partial solution to the toxicity problem but may be limited by myelosuppression. This could be overcome by the use of haematopoietic growth factors, although so far this approach in ovarian cancer is experimental and is limited by the lack of growth factors for platelet production.

Interferon

A number of small phase II studies provide limited evidence of activity of interferon on advanced tumours which are resistant to conventional therapy. In these studies interferon has been administered conventionally (Einhorn et al 1988) and intraperitoneally (Freedman et al 1983) and a small proportion of remissions have been reported. In addition, there is evidence that interferon may be more effective in achieving complete responses in patients with minimal residual disease (Pujade-Lauraine et al 1992). Thus, there is currently considerable interest in using interferon to maintain the complete remissions gained by treatment with chemotherapy. This approach is being investigated in the UK by the Yorkshire Regional Cancer Organization and the North Trent Gynaecological Oncology Group. In this study patients who have responded to conventional cytotoxic chemotherapy are randomized either to observation alone or to receive interferon α given by subcutaneous injection three times a week. The study aims to recruit 400 patients and should help to determine whether interferon increases overall survival in those who achieve complete remission with conventional cytotoxic agents.

Taxol

The management of patients who have failed treatment with cisplatin and/or carboplatin is a major problem. Although some patients who relapse after a long disease-free interval may respond to re-challange with a platinum-based drug, such patients are in the minority. For the majority there is rarely any benefit from the secondary used of conventional cytotoxic agents. Recently, Taxol, a new cytotoxic agent which promotes the assembly and stability of microtubules and is hence a potent inhibitor of mitosis, has shown some promise for patients who have failed on platinum-based chemotherapy. Taxol is derived from the bark of the protected Pacific yew tree and so is in extremely short supply; consequently a relatively small number of patients have been treated with the drug.

A number of phase II studies have been published (Thigpen et al 1990, McGuire et al 1989, Einzig et al 1990) which report responses in approximately one-third of patients who relapsed following conventional chemotherapy. This low response rate has been the subject of a challenging and thought-provoking article by Granai (1992), who rightly questions the media attention given to Taxol, and cautions against exaggerating its benefits, which are unproven and still under study. It is nevertheless an encouraging result in a group of patients in whom response of any sort is a rare event. Attempts to increase the response rate by using high doses of G-CSF were recently reported with 19 out of 38 patients showing objective responses (Sarosy et al 1992).

With such suggested activity in those who have failed on conventional treatment, it is surprising that very few studies have investigated Taxol as a first-line treatment. Those phase I studies which have done so have shown that when given in combination with cisplatin, Taxol should be administered first, otherwise there is marked toxicity resulting from reduced Taxol clearance (Rowinsky et al 1991). Further clinical trials are ongoing.

Preliminary laboratory studies of taxotere, a semi-synthetic drug extracted from the leaves of the English yew tree and therefore in less scarce supply, have suggested that it may have equivalent activity (Alberts et al 1992). It is therefore to be hoped that problems of drug supply will be surmounted and reasonably sized randomized trials will be initiated in the near future. Until such trials are completed there is no evidence whether or not Taxol improves survival in advanced ovarian cancer patients.

Adjuvant hormone therapy

In the past it has been suggested that the use of hormone replacement therapy might give rise to a slight increase in the risk of developing ovarian cancer (Cramer et al 1893). However, it has also been argued that no such association had been established and that such treatment could be used to relieve unpleasant menopausal symptoms in ovarian cancer patients, and furthermore that its use may reduce the risk of osteoporosis and coronary artery disease.

A recent study (Eeles et al 1991) which reported on 373 women under the age of 50 who had had both ovaries removed as part of their ovarian cancer treatment suggested that adjuvant hormone therapy (AHT) might actually improve overall survival in such patients by 12%. However, the reported trend in favour of AHT was not statistically significant and it is therefore not yet clear whether AHT does in fact improve survival. To resolve this problem, a trial has been initiated by the London Gynaecological Oncology Group with the endorsement of the UK Coordination Committee on Cancer Research (UKCCCR). In this trial ovarian cancer patients who have had bilateral oophorectomy are randomized either to receive or not to receive AHT in addition to standard management. Even if this study does not show a significant increase in survival but has equivocal results, it may indicate that AHT can be used to improve the overall quality of life of these patients.

IMPLICATIONS FOR CLINICAL PRACTICE – WHERE NOW?

In a bid to keep abreast of developments in the treatment of advanced ovarian cancer, the practising clinician reading this chapter must inevitably ask 'Do I need to change my current clinical practice as a result of this?' It is now widely recognized that clinical practice should develop on the basis of the results of well-controlled randomized clinical trials, and much of this chapter refers to ongoing clinical research. It is recommended that all advanced ovarian cancer patients should be considered for entry to such trials. This view is supported by the UK Department of Health in that their document on the management of ovarian cancer (Current Clinical Practices 1991) states that 'For the foreseeable future it should be regarded not only as acceptable but *good* practice to enter patients receiving drug or other ancillary therapies for ovarian carcinoma in controlled randomized clinical trials'.

Previous research in advanced ovarian cancer has tended to be rather haphazard, many different drugs, regimens and treatment schedules having been tested against each other in trials that have been too small to give reliable results. Encouragingly, current research appears to be better organized with both national and international collaboration involved in the large multicentre randomized trials previously described.

These modern clinical trials such as icon-2 have been designed to make patient entry as simple as possible and demand little of the clinician in excess of normal clinical practice. Heavy clinical workloads are not disrupted and the patient receives a high standard of treatment and care. Further, it is often not even necessary to choose between one trial and another because the same patient can be entered into more than one study. For example, patients entered into the icon-2 trial are receiving 'standard' treatments and are also eligible for the AHT trial. In this particular case both randomizations can be effected by a single telephone call. The interferon could be considered for patients who achieve remission, and none of the above trials should prevent entry of patients into experimental phase I or II trials if they fail current therapies.

This more scientific approach to both practice and research can only be of benefit to present and future patients and to the profession as a whole.

KEY POINTS FOR CLINICAL PRACTICE

1. The AOCO and the CAP/CP overview have suggested that the treatment of choice for advanced ovarian cancer patients is either CAP or carboplatin given in adequate dose.

2. Patients should be entered into the icon-2 trial to answer the above question.

3. There is no good evidence that increased dose intensity improves survival and considerably more investigation is needed before recommendations can be made for standard clinical practice.

4. Interferon may have a part to play in maintaining remissions, but this can only be decided by ongoing and future randomized clinical trials.

5. AHT may have a role to play in improving survival or quality of life but this must also be determined by current randomized clinical trials.

6. Taxol is a promising new cytotoxic agent, but its place in disease management has yet to be determined by phase I, II and randomized trials.

7. The good forward-thinking clinician tries to enter all his or her ovarian cancer patients into clinical trials.

ACKNOWLEDGEMENTS

We thank Mahesh Parmar, David Machin and David Girling for comments on the manuscript.

REFERENCES

Advanced Ovarian Cancer Trialists Group 1991 Chemotherapy in advanced ovarian cancer: an overview of randomised clinical trials. Br Med J 303: 884–893

Alberts D S, Garcia D, Fanta P et al 1992 Comparative cytotoxicities of taxol and taxotere in vitro against fresh human ovarian cancers. Proc ASCO II Abstract 719: 226

Brodovsky H S, Bauer M, Horton J, Elson P J 1984 Comparison of melphalan with cyclophosphamide, methotrexate and 5-fluorouracil in patients with ovarian cancer. Cancer 53: 844–852

Calvert A H, Newell D R, Gumbrell L A et al 1989 Carboplatin dosage: prospective evaluation of a simple formula based on renal function. J Clin Oncol 3: 1445–1447

Cramer D W, Hutchison G B, Welch W R et al 1983 Determinants of ovarian cancer risk. 1. Reproductive experience and family history. J Natl Cancer Inst 71: 711–716

Eeles R A, Tan S, Wiltshaw E et al 1991 Hormone replacement therapy and survival after surgery for ovarian cancer. Br Med J 302: 259–262

Einhorn N, Ling P, Einhorn S, Strander H 1988 A phase II study of escalating interferon doses in advanced ovarian carcinoma. Am J Clin Oncol 11: 3–6

Einzig A L, Wiernik P H, Sasloff J et al 1990 Phase II study of taxol in patients with advanced ovarian cancer. Proc AACR 31: 187 Abstract 114

Freedman L S 1983 Tables of the number of patients required in clinical trials using the logrank test. Statistics in Medicine 1: 121–129

Granai C O 1992 Ovarian Cancer: unrealistic expectations. N Engl J Med 327: 197–199

Kaye S B, Lewis C R, Paul J et al 1992 Randomised study of two doses of cisplatin with cyclophosphamide in epithelial ovarian cancer. The Lancet 340: 329–333

Levin L, Hryniuk W M 1987 Dose intensity analysis of chemotherapy regimens in ovarian cancer. J Clin Oncol 5: 756–767

McGuire W P, Rowinski E K, Rosenhein N B et al 1989 Taxol: a unique antineoplastic agent with significant activity in advanced epithelial ovarian neoplasms. Ann Int Med 111: 273–279

McGuire W P, Hoskins W J, Brady M F et al 1992 A phase III trial of dose intense versus standard dose cisplatin and cytoxan in advanced ovarian cancer. Proc ASCO II, Abstract 718: 226

MRC Gynaecological Cancer Working Party 1990 An overview in the treatment of advanced ovarian cancer. Br J Cancer 61: 495–496

Ovarian Cancer Meta-Analysis Project (1991) CP versus CAP chemotherapy of ovarian carcinoma: a meta-analysis. J Clin Oncol 9: 1669–1674

Parkin D M, Laara E, Muir C S 1980 Estimates of the world-wide frequency of sixteen major cancers in 1980. Int J Cancer 41: 184–197

Pujade-Lauraine E, Gustella J P, Colombo N et al 1992 Intraperitoneal recombinant human interferon gamma in residual ovarian cancer: efficiency is independent of previous response to chemotherapy. Proc ASCO 11: 225 Abstract 713

Rowinsky E K, Filberts M R, McGuire W P et al 1991 Sequence of taxol and cisplatin: a phase I and pharmacologic study. J Clin Oncol 9: 1692–1703

Sarosy G, Kohn E, Link C et al 1992 Taxol dose intensification in patients with recurrent ovarian cancer. Proc ASCO 11: 226 Abstract 716

Slevin M L, Stubbs L, Plant H J et al 1990 Attitudes to chemotherapy: comparing views of patients with cancer with those of doctors, nurses and general public. Br Med J 300: 1458–1460

Thigpen T, Blessing J, Ball H et al 1990 Phase II trial of taxol as second-line therapy for ovarian carcinoma: a Gynecologic Oncology Group study. Proc ASCO 9: 156 Abstract 604

Whitehouse J M A 1989 Best documented practice. Br Med J 298: 1536

Williams C 1992 Ovarian and cervical cancer. Br Med J 304: 1501–1504

Wiltshaw E, Kroner T 1976 Phase II study of cisdichlorodiammineplatinum (II) (NSC 119875). Cancer Treat Rep 60: 55–60

Wiltshaw E, Evans B, Rustin G et al 1986 A prospective randomised trial comparing high-dose cisplatin with low-dose cisplatin and chlorambucil in advanced ovarian carcinoma. J Clin Oncol 4: 722–729

Young R C, Chabner B A, Hubbard S P et al 1978 Advanced ovarian carcinoma: a prospective clinical trial of melphalan (L-PAM) versus combination chemotherapy. N Engl J Med 299: 1261–1266

12

Endometrial cancer: surgical staging and radical surgery

R. C. Boronow

At the December 1988 National Conference in Los Angeles sponsored by the American Cancer Society, Hervy Averette and I had the privilege of being the 'token gynecologists' on the program. My topic was 'Advances in Diagnosis, Staging, and Management of Low Stage Cervical and Endometrial Cancer' (Boronow 1990).

For background information I had prepared and mailed a survey to all gynecologists who are members of the Society of Gynecological Oncologists regarding their views on the broad aspects of the topic. When it came to tabulating responses both for staging and management for endometrial cancer, the role of surgical staging far and away had the most votes in both categories. Surgical pathologic data that had been developed from studies particularly in the last few decades and their role with prognostic implications are only now beginning to fall into place in a reasonably reproducible way. Indeed, also in 1988, FIGO introduced its 'new' surgical staging for endometrial cancer.

In a very brief way, and clearly from my own personal perspective, I would like to review the last four to five decades of evolving concepts about staging and management of endometrial carcinoma, the most frequent of all invasive gynecologic cancers in the USA. I will review our progress to date, comment on the new staging system and conclude with some speculative remarks. And in the context of the theme, I will weave some definitions of the word 'radical' gleaned from Webster's Dictionary (1989) (Table 12.1).

Table 12.1 Webster's definitions of radical, adj.

1.	of, relating to, or proceeding from a root, as . . . (d) designed to remove the root of a disease or all diseased tissue (as with surgery).
2.	of or relating to the origin: fundamental.
3(b).	tending or disposed to make extreme changes in existing views, habits, conditions or institutions.

Reproduced with permission from *Webster's Ninth New Collegiate Dictionary* . © 1989 by Merriam-Webster Inc., publisher of the Merriam-Webster® dictionaries.

EVOLUTION OF STAGING

Many of us grew up with the international staging system of 1951–1961. This was a modification of the original international staging system, and Dr Brunschwig, my old Chief at Memorial, used to refer to it as the 'League of Nations' staging system (Table 12.2A). The non-operable group was quite sizeable a generation ago, for these were the days before blood banks, modern anesthesia and medical support. From group 2, 'bad operative risks', clinicians recognized that a modest group of patients could be salvaged with intrauterine radium packing only; and this observation gave rise to the clinical practice of combining preoperative uterine, then later uterine–vaginal, radium as an adjunct to be followed by surgery. A further observation of the 'operation advisable' cases came from clinical and pathologic correlations. Some patients relapsed distally whereas others relapsed in the pelvis. On review, many cases involving the lower uterine segment or cervix seemed to incur a high rate of pelvic relapse. Those high in the fundus more often relapsed distally.

This observation was built into the next step in the evolution of FIGO staging (Table 12.2B). Disease confined to the uterus was separated into stage I (corpus only) and stage II (corpus and the cervix). Stages III and IV bear little additional comment.

Table 12.2 Evolution of endometrial cancer staging

A. *Staging 1951–1961*

STAGE 0	Cases which the pathologist considers most likely to be of carcinomatous nature though it is impossible to arrive at a definite microscopic diagnosis
STAGE I	The growth is confined to the uterus
Group 1	Operation advisable
Group 2	Bad operative risk
STAGE II	The growth has spread outside the uterus

B. *Staging 1961–1971*

STAGE 0	Histological findings are suspicious of malignancy but not proven
STAGE I	The carcinoma is confined to the corpus
STAGE II	The carcinoma has involved the corpus and the cervix
STAGE III	The carcinoma has extended outside the uterus but not outside the pelvis
STAGE IV	The carcinoma has extended outside the true pelvis or has obviously involved the mucosa of the bladder or rectum

C. *1971 modifications of stage I*

STAGE I	The carcinoma is confined to the corpus
Stage IA	The length of the uterine cavity is 8 cm or less
Stage IB	The length of the uterine cavity is more than 8 cm

The stage I cases should be subgrouped with regard to the histological type of the adenocarcinoma as follows:

G.1:	highly differentiated adenomatous carcinomas
G.2:	differentiated adenomatous carcinomas with partly solid areas
G.3:	predominantly solid or entirely undifferentiated carcinomas

---

Reproduced with permission from FIGO Annual Reports.

In 1971 a further modification was introduced by FIGO (Table 12.2C). At that point we were advised to divide stage I into IA and IB based on depth of the uterine cavity; and a further important refinement recognized the biological significance of varying degrees of histologic differentiation of the cancer.

CLINICAL MYTHS

In 1975 I had the great privilege of the podium during the 'Parade of Professors' segment at the annual meeting of the American College in Boston. At that time I discussed four statements which I called 'myths', feeling that for the most part there was a widespread view that these statements represented current 'truths' and had to date, in my view, impaired our progress in developing a better understanding of the behaviour of endometrial cancer (Boronow 1976). The first 'myth' was that endometrial cancer was a benign disease. I had generated a bar graph which reflected the then current results both as reported in the Annual Report and a review of seven contemporary series collected by Paul Morrow. The striking observation was that stage-for-stage 5-year survival for endometrial cancer was essentially identical to 5-year survival stage-for-stage for carcinoma of the cervix, which most people felt was a much more virulent disease. Clearly, neither were benign diseases! The overall results of all endometrial cancer cases treated was better than overall results for cervical cancer, but that was merely a reflection of the fact that approximately 75% of corpus cancer cases were seen in the stage I setting.

The second 'myth' was that the prognostic factors had been sufficiently defined. I called the unfavourable prognostic factors 'predisposing factors for extrauterine spread'. These factors included lower uterine segment (isthmus and cervix); less favourable histology (poor and moderately differentiated tumors); and significant myometrial invasion (deep — outer one-third; and intermediate — middle one-third). These factors had been discussed in our literature and were often referred to as 'virulence factors'. But it is apparent that with treatment directed at the uterus, when relapse occurs we can presume, so to speak, that 'the rats were out of the barn before the barn was burned down'. We can assess whether upper or lower pole is involved preoperatively and we can assess histologic grade. What we cannot assess preoperatively is depth of myometrial invasion (until the advent of high-tech — and, I must add, high-cost — imaging techniques of dubious merit, in my view).

So we as clinicians generally have made inferences over recent decades to guide us in our selection of therapy. You have heard the dialogue many times: 'Well, it is a well-differentiated cancer and the uterus is small. I think I'll just take it out!' For the well-differentiated cancers, most are confined to the endometrium or have superficial invasion. But 10–15% have significant myometrial invasion and the overall 5-year salvage for grade 1 in the literature is 85–95%. Those tumors of intermediate differentiation again are relatively superficial for the most part, but an increasing percentage (15–20%) have more significant myometrial invasion, and the worldwide literature reports a 70–85% grade 2 salvage for stage I endometrial cancer. For grade 3 cancers, however, about half are found to have significant myometrial invasion, and grade 3 salvage in the literature was generally in the 50–60% range, and only occasionally a bit higher.

Credit must be given to Alan Ng, James Reagan, and Budd Wentz at Case Western Reserve. They were the most vigorous to correlate survival by grade and myometrial invasion. They used the Broder's grade of histologic differentiation (four grades) and a modified Duke's classification for invasion. From an early report (Kistner et al 1973) they demonstrated, for example, that for grade 2 cancers, if disease was confined to the endometrium only, there was a 93% 5-year cure rate, but for this same histologic grade, once deep myometrial invasion is reached, the 5-year survival was 38%. Further, for depth of invasion, they demonstrated that for group B cases (disease confined to the inner half of the myometrium) there was an 87% 5-year cure for grade 1 cases, but a 50% 5-year cure for histologic grade 3 and 4 cases.

The third 'myth' was that the best way to treat endometrial cancer had been defined. For those whose memories allow reflection on three and four decades ago, they will appreciate that there were probably more different ways to treat stages I and II endometrial cancer, from institution to institution, than with approaches to the other common gynecologic malignancies. We all did what we were taught to do in our residency programs and we typified the words of Alexander Brunschwig, who would admonish us: 'Doctor, you're just a product of your training!'

There were those who favored surgery only. There were those who favored a preoperative radium packing. And there were a small number who believed that all patients should receive pelvic external beam therapy preoperatively. Those of us who came through Northwestern University Medical School in the 1950s and early 1960s recall the differences of approach taken by the Chief at Chicago Wesley (George Gardner MD), the Chief at Passavant Memorial (John Brewer MD) and the Chief at Evanston (David Danforth MD). Dr Gardner was the overall Department Chairman and he believed in primary surgery. Dr Brewer favored routine preop radium packing. My Chief at Evanston, Dr Danforth, would usually call his residency days room-mate, Dr Saul Gusberg, and get his advice. No wonder the clinical schizophrenia of those of us emerging from the Northwestern system! When I embarked on my personally defined program of post-residency training years, I got the approval of Dr Brunschwig at Memorial and then Dr Rutledge at the M. D. Anderson to review all of the endometrial cancer at the institution treated during the tenure of each of these men. In my naivety I was convinced that by comparing results achieved by one institution that relied heavily on a radical surgical approach with the other institution that relied heavily on adjuvant radiation therapy, clearly some significant differences would emerge. Table 12.3 from

Table 12.3   Endometrial cancer results at two major centers

	M. D. Anderson Hospital[a] (1948–1963)		Memorial Hospital[b] (1949–1965)	
	No. of patients	5-year survical (%)	No. of patients	5-year survival (%)
Stage I	270	77	539	74
Stage II				
Clinical	19	58	24	54
Biopsy	44	61	(occult)[c] 68	57

Reproduced with permission from Boronow (1973).
[a]Data from Boronow (1969b).
[b]Data from Homesley et al (1976).
[c]Clinical stage I cases with cervical spread determined by pathologist.

an earlier publication demonstrates, however, that for stage I disease and for stage II clinical versus occult or microscopic there was in fact no statistically significant difference between the outcome of patients treated at these two institutions with rather different management philosophies! It thus became apparent to me that the era of comparing inter-institutional results had to be relegated to a thing of the past and that prospective studies are necessary.

The final 'myth' was that pelvic and periaortic nodes were of little or no consequence in endometrial cancer. There had been a number of reports in the literature, beginning with Javert, Meigs, Parsons, Brunschwig and others, about pelvic node metastasis (Table 12.4A). The formal radical abdominal hysterectomy and pelvic lymphadenectomy with en bloc resection of the parametrial tissues was enthusiastically advocated by a few surgeons in the past. This is the first definition of 'radical' (Table 12.1) to consider. When applied in a relatively unselected manner, no increase in salvage rate was evident. In addition, the patient population with endometrial cancer is considerably less favorable for this operation than those with cervical cancer, the group for which this operation has its greatest application. Certainly, however, when the cervix is involved, this procedure may be selectively applied. The earlier critical review of this topic by Rutledge (1974) remains a classic reference. Thus, the failure to demonstrate improved survival, and the necropsy data that had been generated from the autopsy table (Table 12.4B) suggesting that if pelvic nodes were involved the aortic nodes would also be involved, so combined to create the widespread sentiment that concern about the status of the pelvic nodes was an idle clinical exercise.

I had contributed to this 'mythology' in several ways. The first was an illustration (Fig. 12.1) that I had generated for a publication on endometrial cancer in the late 1960s (Boronow 1969a). This demonstrated the dual lymphatics of the uterus that parallel the dual vasculature of the uterus. The clinical implication is that disease in the body of the uterus drains by way of

Table 12.4   Lymph node metastasis in endometrial cancer

Reference	Total no.	Positive nodes	
		No.	%
A. Clinical incidence			
Randall (1950)	20	4	20.0
Javert (1952)	50	14	28.8
Brunschwig & Murphy (1954)	57	10	17.5
Peightal (1954)	23	4	17.4
Liu & Meigs (1955)	47	11	23.4
Kottmeier & Moberger (1955)	163	7	4.3
Lefevre (1956)	45	7	15.6
Roberts (1961)	22	5	22.8
Barber (1962)	277	59	21.3
Miller (1962)	21	3	14.3
Alford (1992)	32	3	9.4
Gusberg & Yannopoulos (1964)	7	0	0.0
Davis (1964)	151	21	13.9
Dobbie (1965)	730	12	1.6
Carmichael & Bean (1967)	128	12	9.4
Lees (1969)	129	17	13.2
B. Autopsy incidence			
Andriezen & Leitch (1906)	33	15	45.5
Henriksen (1949)	64	47	73.4
Bunker (1959)	44	22	50.0
Beck & Latour (1963)	36	25	69.4

Modified with permission from Plentl and Friedman (1971).

the ovarian vessels and directly to the aortic retroperitoneum, whereas disease involving the lower segment of the uterus and the cervix picks up the hypogastric system of lymphatics, thereby draining to the pelvic nodes.

My second contribution to this 'mythology' was my review from the M. D. Anderson that supported this notion. We published a paper in which none of 71 node-dissected stage I cases were found to have pelvic node metastasis (Boronow 1969b).

SURGICAL STAGING EMERGENCE

The major impetus to surgical staging in endometrial cancer came from the Oxford work of Sir John Stallworthy and collaborators, who in 1970 and 1971 published several papers (Lewis et al 1970, Stallworthy 1971) reflecting a 20-year experience with the Wertheim hysterectomy and lymphadenectomy in early-stage endometrial cancer. During that time span they had operated on 109 patients and the results shocked the American reader. In stage I endometrial cancer, Lewis et al (1970) reported a 5.5% incidence of pelvic node metastasis in grade 1 cancers, 10% for grade 2 and an astonishing 26% for grade 3. When there was no myometrial invasion or invasion of up to 2 mm, there was no pelvic node metastasis, but beyond 2 mm of invasion the incidence of pelvic nodes was 24%. Furthermore, when external beam

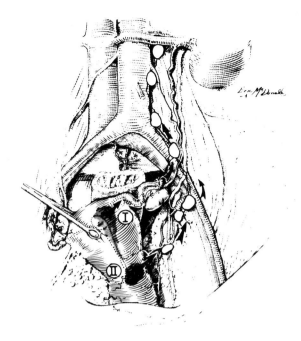

Fig. 12.1 Dual lymphatic drainage of uterus. Stage I endometrial cancer (I) drains via the infundibulopelvic ligament, primarily to nodes above the pelvic brim and retroperitoneal aortic nodes. Stage II endometrial cancer is extension to involve both corpus and cervix (II) and drains primarily via the pericervical lymphatics to the pelvic nodes. Reproduced with permission from Boronow (1969a).

therapy was given to the pelvis to patients with the findings of pelvic node metastasis, over one-third (36%) of these patients achieved 5-year survival.

This prompted a review by Morrow (Morrow et al 1973) of available literature. Very little could be found on the outcome of patients with pelvic node metastasis, but he did find that among 25 patients reported 10 (40%) were 5-year survivors. Paul Morrow and I were discussing the Oxford report and my review of the M. D. Anderson experience (Boronow 1969b), and we concluded that there was no rational way to explain the irreconcilable differences between these two reports. We agreed at that time to develop a two-institution study, for we had a reasonably good clinical volume to investigate. I had been at the University of Mississippi for 4 years. Paul and Phil DiSaia were just beginning a program at Southern California. However, Bill Creasman had just moved to Duke, so we invited his participation, and this three-institution study soon gained approval from the Gynecologic Oncology Group as 'Pilot Study 1', thereby providing funding for data analysis and the like.

Our surgical study protocol was not a 'radical' hysterectomy on these patients, but rather a conservative extrafascial hysterectomy, and then move laterally to the retroperitoneum to dissect the pelvic nodes and to liberally sample the periaortic chain. We left the parametria and the ureters undisturbed, thereby minimizing morbidity.

Yet our purpose embodied the second definition of 'radical' (Table 12.1). We proposed to collect a prospective histologic database of uterus, tubes, ovaries and lymph nodes upon which further studies might be envisaged. This seemed not only an appropriate but also a desirable definition of 'radical'. We hoped that cases not requiring any further treatment could be more precisely identified. And we wondered if patients at high risk for relapse could be identified more precisely; then we would add external beam therapy to treat only those at risk, thereby avoiding treatment for the majority of patients not at risk. The final analysis of the clinical–pathologic features of our 222 cases in the pilot study was published in 1984 (Boronow et al 1984). The risk factors and the recurrence patterns were published the following year (DiSaia et al 1985). The results of our pilot study, the later expanded GOG study (Creasman et al 1987), and the original Oxford report (Lewis et al 1970) were strikingly similar.

Several speculations emerged from these earlier studies. We (Boronow 1976) contrasted the Oxford report (1970) of pelvic node metastasis by grade, with Cheon's report (1969) indicating the percentage of cases with significant myometrial invasion for each of the three grades. The comparative plotting of these two sets of data suggested the first speculation: that with significant myometrial invasion the patient might have an approximately 50% risk of lymph node metastasis irrespective of grade!

Table 12.5 (data from our 1984 report) breaks down the actual risk of pelvic node metastasis for each grade by the four categories of invasion that we defined: for endometrial disease only there was virtually no risk of pelvic node metastasis, irrespective of histologic grade; for tumors infiltrating the inner third of the myometrium the risk was substantial for grade 3; for tumors infiltrating the middle third of the myometrium the risk of node metastasis was substantial for grades 2 and 3. And for tumors infiltrating the outer third of the myometrium the risk was substantial for all grades. Admittedly when broken down into individual subsets the numbers were small. Nevertheless, the data suggested a usable algorithm for an intraoperative frozen section decision to dissect pelvic nodes, and having a reasonable likelihood of finding metastatic disease: for endometrium only (all histologic grades) the risk was negligible; for superficial myometrial invasion the risk was substantial only for grade 3; for middle third invasion the risk was substantial for grades 2 and 3. And for deep myometrial invasion all grades of tumor had substantial risk. So the risk was not precisely 50% as initially speculated, but was indeed significant (20–45%).

We further incorporated features such as vascular space involvement, spread to the lower uterine segment or adnexae and the various cell types. Our cases broke down quite neatly into two groups: the negligible risk of node metastasis (0–4%) and the substantial risk of node metastasis (20–45%) (Table

Table 12.5 Node metastasis by maximum invasion and grade

Depth and grade	Total cases	Pelvic nodes		Aortic nodes			
		Number	%	Total nodes sampled	Total found positive	% sampled nodes positive	% total cases positive
FIGO stage I							
Endometrium							
Grade 1	58	1	1.7	47	1	2.1	1.7
Grade 2	27	1	3.7	15	0	0.0	0.0
Grade 3	7	0	0.0	6	0	0.0	0.0
Superficial							
Grade 1	27	0	0.0	18	0	0.0	0.0
Grade 2	40	1	2.5	26	0	0.0	0.0
Grade 3	13	3	23.1	11	5	45.5	38.5
Intermediate							
Grade 1	4	0	0.0	2	0	0.0	0.0
Grade 2	8	2	25.5	4	1	25.0	12.5
Grade 3	5	1	20.0	3	0	0.0	0.0
Deep							
Grade 1	4	1	25.0	3	0	0.0	0.0
Grade 2	13	6	46.2	9	5	55.5	38.5
Grade 3	16	7	43.7	14	5	35.7	31.3
Total	222	23	10.4	157	17	10.8	7.6

Reproduced with permission from Boronow et al (1984).

12.6). The 'negligible risk' for node metastasis group represented about 75% of the case material, and approximately 25% were in the 'substantial risk' category for node metastasis. In late 1988 FIGO incorporated some of this type of material into a revised Corpus Staging System that is now *Surgical Staging*. This topic will be discussed further.

The other speculation, or rhetorical question, suggested by the prevailing views of the time was: 'pelvic node metastasis always meant aortic node metastasis'. In our preliminary evaluation of 74 cases we found that when the pelvic nodes were dissected and were negative, the finding of aortic node metastasis was documented in only one case (1.5%). Conversely, when pelvic node metastasis was documented, the risk of aortic node metastasis was 60% (Boronow 1976). This was fascinating in the context of the Oxford report (Lewis et al 1970) where one-third of patients with positive pelvic nodes were salvaged with the addition of pelvic radiation therapy. That suggests, at least to me, that the addition of pelvic radiation therapy was adequate to control occult disease in the pelvis, and further, that this group of one-third salvaged did not have spread beyond the field of radiation therapy treatment; and conversely, that the two-thirds of patients who were not salvaged by postoperative radiation therapy to the pelvic volume must indeed have had aortic node spread. Evaluation of our preliminary data lends credence to that

Table 12.6   Risk features for
node metastasis

A. *Negligible risk*
Invasion of myometrium
    Endometrium only, grades 1, 2 and
3
    Inner, grades 1 and 2
    Middle one-third, grade 1
Vascular space involvement (VSI)
    None
Occult spread to cervix and/or adnexa
    None
Cell type
    Adenocarcinoma (AC)
    Adenocanthoma (AA)

B. *Substantial risk*
Invasion of myometrium
    Inner one-third, grade 3
    Middle one-third, grades 2 and 3
    Outer one-third, grades 1, 2 and 3
Vascular space involvement (VSI)
    Present
Occult spread to cervix and/or adnexa
    Present
Cell type
    Adenosquamous (AS)
    Papillary serous (UPSC)
    Clear cell (CC)

Modified from Boronow (1987) and
Boronow et al (1984).

hypothesis. A review of the our full 222 cases again demonstrated essentially the same thing. Specifically, when pelvic node metastasis was not found, the incidence of aortic node metastasis was on the order of 2%, but when pelvic node metastasis was found the risk of aortic node metastasis (among sampled cases) was 60.9% (Boronow et al 1984).

THE NEW FIGO STAGING SYSTEM

The challenge, of course, to surgical staging is that if we discover poor prognostic feature(s), can we do anything about it? Before we pursue this topic, I would like to digress for a moment to comment on what I believe to be an unfortunate development handed down to us from FIGO in the name of 'progress' (Table 12.7). Indeed I believe this 'extreme' change is both unnecessary and abusively 'radical' (the last definition in Table 12.1).

I have two criticisms of the new system. The first is that I believe that despite the effort to be more precise, the system is nevertheless riddled with imprecision and flaws; the second is that it is dangerously meddlesome.

With regard to the first issue, I can allocate any given case to any given staging system for purposes of record keeping. I see four to five new

Table 12.7 Surgical staging of carcinoma of the corpus uteri

The FIGO Committee on Gynecology Oncology agreed upon the system for surgical staging for carcinoma of the corpus uteri at the meeting in Rio de Janeiro in October 1988.

Definitions of the surgical stages in carcinoma of the corpus uteri

Stage IA	Grade 1,2,3	Tumor limited to endometrium
Stage IB	Grade 1,2,3	Invasion to $< \frac{1}{2}$ myometrium
Stage IC	Grade 1,2,3	Invasion $\geqslant \frac{1}{2}$ myometrium
Stage IIA	Grade 1,2,3	Endocervical glandular involvement only
Stage IIB	Grade 1,2,3	Cervical stromal invasion
Stage IIIA	Grade 1,2,3	Tumor invades serosa and/or adnexae and/or positive peritoneal cytology
Stage IIIB	Grade 1,2,3	Vaginal metastases
Stage IIIC	Grade 1,2,3	Metastases to pelvic and/or para-aortic lymph nodes
Stage IVA	Grade 1,2,3	Tumor invasion of bladder and/or bowel mucosa
Stage IVB		Distant metastases including intra-abdominal and/or inguinal lymph node

Histopathology: degree of differentiation
Cases of carcinoma of the corpus should be grouped with regard to the degree of differentiation of the adenocarcinoma as follows:

G1:   5% or less of a non-squamous or non-morular solid growth pattern
G2:   6–50% of a non-squamous or non-morular solid growth pattern
G3:   More than 50% of a non-squamous or non-morular solid growth pattern

Notes on pathological grading

1. Notable nuclear atypia, inappropriate for the architectural grade, raises the grade of a grade 1 or grade 2 tumor by 1
2. In serous adenocarcinomas, clear cell adenocarcinomas and squamous cell carcinomas, nuclear grading takes precedence
3. Adenocarcinomas with squamous differentiation are graded according to the nuclear grade of the glandular component

---

Reproduced with permission from Pettersson (1991).

endometrial cancer cases per month in my referral practice, so record keeping is not a chore. But in my view this new system is not at all helpful. The first purpose of staging (irrespective of disease of anatomic setting) is to provide a common language — a worldwide uniformity to the clinical vocabulary — by which data from various sources maybe reviewed and compared. Inherent in the concept of 'staging' (as originally defined) is the relationship of progressive staging to progressive anatomic extent of disease, and this should reasonably reflect prognostic groups in a progressively less favourable fashion. I am not convinced that the current recommendations necessarily follow this principle.

I have only a few problems with the stages I and II revision. Since most of our experience, at least in the USA with assessing myometrial invasion, involved four groups — endometrium only, inner third of myometrium, middle third of myometrium, outer third (rather than inner half and outer half) — I would have preferred four groups rather than three, or IA–ID rather than IA–IC. While this criticism is 'fine tuning' rather than a 'flaw', I think all will agree that the outcome in stage IIA G1 cases is undoubtedly better than for stage IC G3 cases. Further, our instructions with clinical staging were 'when it is doubtful to which stage a particular case should be allotted, the case must be referred to the earlier stage'. Obviously, with surgical staging, the case is allotted to the highest stage, based on the most extreme finding.

Stages III and IV give me more problems, however. Stage III is remarkably contrived. Serosal invasion is, in my view (and most with whom I have talked) the extreme of deep myometrial invasion of stage I disease. And it is quite a different entity from adnexal spread. Those two represent very different features and should not be grouped together. Indeed the FIGO committee contradicts itself: surface disease of the uterus is 'stage III' whereas surface diseases of the ovary (in the ovarian staging system) may be 'stage I'. The latter seems appropriate and the former does not. Also, positive cytology should be separate as it is with ovarian cancer. In my experience vaginal metastais, stage IIIB (as a single variant), has a better prognosis than adnexal spread, stage IIIA. Pelvic node metastasis has a better prognosis than aortic node metastasis, and again these two findings should be separated, not grouped together. The 'and/or' in stage IVB is confusing. As written, one would wonder if this is intra-abdominal (aortic) *nodes* and/or inguinal *nodes* (if so, this duplicates stage IIIC). I suspect this means intra-abdominal spread, as parietal or visceral peritoneal spread, such as cul de sac implants, omental metastasis and the like, but this is not clear as currently written.

In 1980 Dr Philip Rubin solicited a series of articles on endometrial cancer for his 'red journal' of radiation oncology. In my contribution I stated then 'What isn't needed is a new staging system for any gynecologic cancer. What is needed is proper use of current systems. And what may be useful is consideration of possible extensions of current systems' (Boronow 1980). We had a clinical staging system that rationally progressed through increasing degrees of anatomic extent of disease. The FIGO Committee had many options to 'fine tune' the previous system within the frame of reference of the pathologic tumor node metastasis (pTNM) options. All the factors currently considered could be worked into the old system. In my view, this was not only a radical change but, more to the point, an unnecessary change.

My second criticism may be the one most worthy of careful consideration. This is the whole issue of whether mandatory surgical staging is desirable or even wise. When Paul Morrow and I envisioned the prospective study of early-stage endometrial cancer to include pelvic lymph node dissection and liberal aortic node sampling, we felt very strongly that the purpose was to gather a sizeable body of clinical pathologic data which would better define high-risk factors for extrauterine spread. At no point in our project, nor in *our* publications, did we recommend routine lymph node dissections as a part of standard therapy. This was a clinical research study.

As already stated, our cases broke down fairly cleanly into two groups of patients. About 25% of our case material had a substantial risk for lymph node metastasis. This 'substantial risk' was on the order of 20–40%. However, about 75% of the patients fell into the so-called negligible risk for node metastasis, i.e. 0–5%. By mandating surgical staging we are clearly suggesting that 75% of the stage I patients be subjected to unnecessary and potentially hazardous lymph node surgery. Two cases of unnecessary lymph node surgery illustrate this point. The first was a lady in her 80s with a well-differentiated endometrial cancer with no appreciable myometrial invasion. The operating obstetrician/gynecologist called in a general surgeon colleague who attempted pelvic and aortic node sampling and in the course of the procedure damaged and repaired one ureter. The patient subsequently developed a fistula, became septic, was in the intensive care unit for a protracted period of time, and ultimately had a nephrectomy. She did survive. The second patient was in her 60s with a well-differentiated endometrial cancer with no myometrial invasion on frozen section. This was done in a teaching institution and a Fellow, without benefit of attending faculty, lacerated the vena cava at the level of its bifurcation. Staff was called, but suturing efforts were to no avail. After about 4 hours a vascular surgeon was called. The patient developed disseminated intravascular coagulopathy (DIC), was given about 40 units of blood, and died in the intensive care unit.

Numerous reports have appeared in the literature attesting to the low morbidity of 'staging' node dissections or node sampling when done by skilled gynecologic oncologists. That is not the issue. Most cases of endometrial cancer are operated by generalists and it is common practice for a general surgeon to be called in to 'do the nodes'. This parceling of care is wrong; and even when done by skilled people, it is still wrong. When will we relearn the great surgical aphorism: 'The *ability* to do an operation must not become the *indication* to do it!'

Evaluation of our original material (Boronow et al 1984) produced a very usable piece of information. In the entire experience, slightly more than one-half of the cases with positive nodes were suspected on gross clinical inspection and palpation, both for pelvic (12 of 23, or 52.2%) and aortic (9 of 17, or 52.9%) node metastasis. Among nodes removed that were not clinically suspicious, the yield of occult metastasis was low: 11 positive of 210 clinically negative pelvic node dissections, or 5.2%, and 8 positive of 148 clinically negative aortic nodes (liberally sampled), or 5.4%. This reality should dampen the enthusiasm for random plucking or 'sampling' clinically negative nodes. Little is likely to be learned, and much damage may be done!

I have no doubt that the current FIGO recommendations represent an effort to be beneficial; but I believe such a radical change was unnecessary and inadvisable. If possible, I suggest that the FIGO Committee seriously reconsider their current recommendations.

PROSPECTS AND SPECULATION

I would like to discuss the challenge of surgical staging or, more precisely, the challenge of the clinical implications of surgical–pathologic data. Table 12.8

Table 12.8 Carcinoma of the uterine corpus: review of the 5-year survival rate by stage reported in volumes 16–20 (1962–1981)

Stage	Patients treated in				
	1962–1968 (Vol.16)	1969–1972 (Vol. 17)	1973–1975 (Vol. 18)	1976–1978 (Vol. 19)	1979–1981 (Vol. 20)
I	71.0	73.6	74.2	75.1	72.3
II	49.7	55.7	57.4	57.8	56.4
III	30.7	31.3	29.2	30.0	31.5
IV	9.3	9.2	9.6	10.6	10.5
Total	63.0	65.4	66.6	67.7	65.1

Reproduced with permission from Pettersson (1989).

is from Volume 20 of the Annual Report and reflects endometrial cancer 5-year survival by stages reported in Volumes 16–20. We have not improved our results over the years studied, 1962–1981. That is precisely why we need to try some different clinical approaches.

For years, we have added whole pelvic radiation therapy to poor-prognosis disease. Over the last four decades whole pelvic radiation therapy has been our gold standard of treatment. An informative study from the Norwegian Radium Hospital (Aadlers et al 1980) provides interesting information. All 540 patients had primary surgery and postoperative vaginal vault radium. The patients were then divided into two groups: group A (277 patients) with no further treatment and group B (263 patients) with postoperative external beam pelvic radiation therapy. In this large group of patients the 5-year survival was essentially the same (91% and 89%, respectively). The death and recurrence rates were essentially the same (12.3% and 11.8%, respectively). With those treated with vaginal radium only, however, the incidence of vaginal pelvic failure was higher (6.9%) than in the group receiving postoperative whole pelvic therapy (1.9%). Conversely, the distant metastasis rate was higher in those treated with pelvic radiation therapy (9.9% versus 5.4%). Evaluation of both the GOG pilot study (DiSaia et al 1985) and the group-wide corpus study made similar observations (Morrow et al 1991).

Regional control is important but total control is more important. These data suggest that pelvic radiation therapy improves control in the pelvis, but contributes nothing to spread beyond the pelvis. This strongly supports the long-established principle of 'metastasis from metastasis'. I firmly believe that when whole pelvic radiation therapy is felt to be indicated the use of extended field radiation therapy is more appropriate, and this has been our practice for several years. Indeed, fragmentary data from many sources support this (Boronow 1991).

Throughout the decade of the 1970s and into the 1980s, the role of surgical staging in cervical cancer and the role of extended field therapy underwent extensive study. High complications and relatively low survival rates brought the technique for advanced cervical cancer to a state of relative disuse. Over two decades of experience with extended field radiation therapy in cancer of the cervix has taught many lessons: the non-curability of bulky aortic disease and the potential for significant morbidity; therefore, the necessity to decrease both daily dose fraction and total dose delivered to the extended field. The data available suggest that if disease can be surgically cleared, if the procedure is done with skill, and if nominal dose fractions are reduced, extended field therapy can be given with relative safety and with a reasonable prospect of control of very low-volume disease.

A couple of reports with cervical cancer are illustrative. The Philadelphia report (Rubin et al 1984) includes a small series of low-stage cervical cancer cases treated by radical hysterectomy with positive aortic nodes excised that achieved a 43% 5-year survival when extended field therapy was added. A Japanese report (Inoue & Morita 1988) included high common iliac nodes as representative of aortic node metastasis, and they reported a 57% 5-year cure with extended field therapy. When the nodes are completely resected, the cure rate was 67% and even with unresected nodes, by boosting the target, 44% achieved 5-year cure. Similarly in low-stage endometrial cancer only a few small series are available. The 3–5-year survival with positive aortic nodes is reported in the 40–60% range (Blythe et al 1986, Feuer & Calanog 1987, Komaki et al 1983, Potish et al 1985, Morrow et al 1991) — certainly impressive and gratifying responses.

Roger Potish, of the University of Minnesota, describes three decision strategies for the use of extended field radiation therapy (Potish et al 1984). Strategy 1 is surgical with application of extended field therapy only to those patients with proven positive aortic nodes. Strategy 3 is a clinical judgment that concludes that the use of extended field therapy is too hazardous and/or of unsatisfactory value; therefore, no patients are treated. The third option (strategy 2) is a clinical strategy in which *all* patients will receive extended field therapy. This is not a new idea. Marvin Rotman and his group in New York had a trial of this experience in the mid 1970s with a definite improvement in cervical cancer stage IIB treated with extended field therapy (Rotman et al 1978). I find this strategy attractive and appropriate for endometrial cancer.

We *have* learned much about the use of extended field therapy. Our personal experience of over 100 patients with endometrial cancer among a total experience of well over 400 patients treated with extended field therapy indicates that this treatment can be given safely with negligible morbidity, and at the dose levels employed provides a reasonably good prospect of occult disease control. Obviously we will not cure all patients treated, but my experience suggests that some of these patients are cured and many more have greater than anticipated protracted intervals of disease control before relapse becomes evident.

OUR CHALLENGE

In a quote attributed to Aristotle 'The whole is more than the sum of the parts'. Indeed, cancer management efficacy must be judged not only by 5-year survival, but also by improved disease-free interval unimpaired by major treatment morbidity.

I believe if we make use of our current clinical–pathologic database in endometrial cancer and if we make use more creatively of the radiotherapy techniques currently available, and also if we consider the utilization of concomitant infusion chemotherapy as a further adjuvant to our therapy treatment planning, we have the opportunity to impact significantly on the survival of patients with poor-prognosis yet low-stage endometrial cancer.

RECOMMENDED PRACTICAL APPROACH TO MANAGEMENT

Figure 12.2 outlines a specific management approach. Approximately 75% of endometrial cancer occurs within the old stage I setting (confined to the body of the uterus), compared with about one-third of the cervical cancer cases. At least another 10% are stage II (cervix and corpus). The observation that the vast majority of cases are 'operable' cases underscores the necessity of careful appreciation of the pathologic variables, both in understanding prognosis and in planning therapy. In the management of each patient there is a significant place for reflection, judgment and individualization.

The prognostic implications of the surgical–pathologic data that have emerged in the last decade or two have been reviewed in the first portion of this chapter. The prognostic implications have fallen into place in a more consistent and reproducible way. Therapeutic implications remain more elusive. New and exciting data — somewhat conflicting — are emerging in the areas of estrogen and progesterone receptors, flow cytometry, ploidy and cellular DNA analysis, and in the search for serum markers. These data have not matured sufficiently to be used to make clinical decisions in patient care. This is particularly true where this information is discordant with the basic clinical–pathologic material at hand.

In general, I prefer to use preoperative cesium treatment, except in grade 1 cancer and in patients of advanced age or with particular medical infirmities, followed by hysterectomy within a week. This approach makes use of the uterus for brachytherapy insertion, permitting a higher parametrial dose to be given more safely, in contrast to using post-hysterectomy colpostats.

The abdomen is opened with a subumbilical midline incision, and pelvic and abdominal peritoneal washings using several hundred milliliters of normal saline are taken *before* any palpation or manipulation of the uterus. The head of the table may be raised and lowered several times to facilitate a thorough lavage. The upper abdomen is then meticulously palpated with attention to peritoneal surfaces, liver, undersurfaces of diaphragm, omentum and the para-aortic region. A generous omental biopsy is taken if the histology has shown uterine papillary serous carcinoma. The intestines are then packed away and the extrafascial hysterectomy with bilateral salpingo-oophorectomy carried out. It is not necessary to excise a generous vaginal cuff, but if the

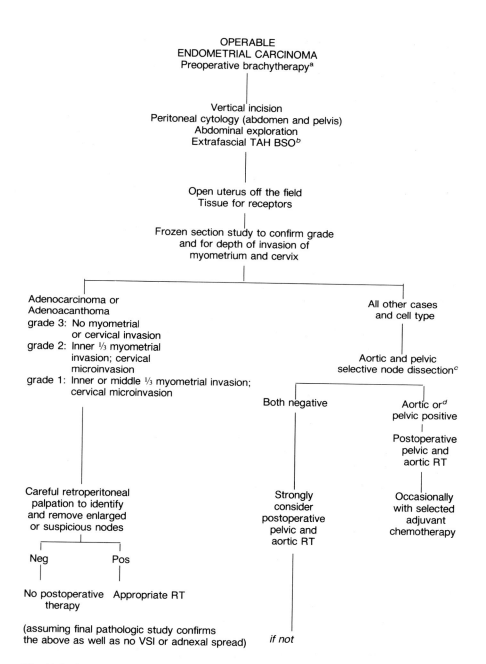

Fig. 12.2 Protocol for management of clinically operative endometrial carcinoma.
[a]Tandem and ovoids (Fletcher) for all but grade 1 cases; 5000 cGy vaginal surface dose
maximum; 4000 cGy to Point A.
[b]Total abdominal hysterectomy, bilateral salpingo-oophorectomy.
[c]Target nodes are removed for frozen section analysis first. If positive, further node dissection
in that area is unnecessary.
[d]If there are multiple or large aortic node metastases, the scalene fat pad may be removed.
Metastasis at that level would be a contraindication to extended field radiation therapy.
RT = radiation therapy; Pos = metastases present; VSI = vascular space invasion; Neg =
metastases absent.

effort is made to excise 1–2 cm of vaginal cuff this will ensure that all the cervix is removed.

Our next steps are guided by frozen section study of the total abdominal hysterectomy-bilateral salpingo oophorectomy (TAH-BSO) specimen and assessment of the patient with the retroperitoneal spaces opened. Any suspicious or clinically positive nodes are excised. As stated previously, approximately 50% of the positive node yield in our GOG pilot study was from nodes that were clinically positive or suspicious on inspection and palpation. Of the nodes removed that were not clinically suspicious, the yield of occult metastasis was low. Therefore, we pursue the clinically negative nodes more vigorously only in the subsets who are more likely at risk.

If no suspicious pelvic nodes are found, the obturator and iliac nodes (external, internal and common) are removed, much less extensively than with a lymphadenectomy as part of radical surgery for cervical cancer. It is a debulking procedure and the vessels are not stripped clean. Adventitial tissue and lateral channels are preserved. All para-aortic nodes are excised that are clinically positive or suspicious on careful palpation after opening the retroperitoneal space, provided this can be done without undue hazard. Further, when massive adenopathy is encountered the diagnosis is confirmed by small biopsy and the procedure is aborted, for such a patient is not salvageable. If nothing suspicious is found, the precaval and aortic fat pad is removed from just below the bifurcation of the vena cava and aorta and upwards along these vessels for 3–4 cm, and occasionally to the level of the renal vessels. A complete retroperitoneal para-aortic dissection is rarely done. The morbidly obese or otherwise medically compromised patient is usually excluded from aortic node sampling. In our pilot study only 157 of the 222 patients had aortic nodes sampled.

If postoperative treatment is indicated, the dual spread pattern should always be treated with routine use of the pelvic and aortic fields (Boronow 1991). We consider this form of therapy routinely when there are other poor prognostic features even in the absence of confirmed nodal metastasis. Finally, we also employ adjuvant chemotherapy in patients with particularly poor prognostic features such as vascular space involvement and positive pelvic nodes and adenosquamous or uterine papillary serous histology. We have not seen side-effects different from that expected with the use of pelvic radiotherapy.

The management of positive peritoneal washings is a very difficult issue. The quantitative aspects of positivity have recently received some attention. Therapy reports have not been controlled. Positive peritoneal cytologic findings in endometrial cancer are frequently a reflection of more advanced disease, as shown by a variety of other single and combined unfavorable pathologic features. The true significance of positive peritoneal cytologic findings remains uncertain. Our therapy bias favors the use of progestational therapy for grade 1 cases. Despite the shortcomings of the published data, it seems reasonable to accept that, at least in the grade 2 and grade 3 lesions with abundant malignant cells in the peritoneal cytology sample, the prognosis for these patients is seriously affected. What action should be taken is uncertain. Intraperitoneal nuclide therapy may be a logical choice in the absence of metastasis or other risk factors. Our lack of enthusiasm for this therapy, however, relates in part to distribution problems and also, primarily, that the vast majority of the beta energy of chromic phosphate is absorbed within the first millimetre of depth from source. Whole-abdomen radiation therapy may be preferable for patients who have additional indications for pelvic and aortic field irradiation. We have utilized this occasionally beginning with whole-abdomen therapy and boosting pelvic and para-aortic volumes with field-within-a-field techniques.

REFERENCES

Aalders J, Abeler V, Kolstad P, Onsrud M 1980 Postoperative external irradiation and prognostic parameters in stage I endometrial carcinoma, clinical and histopathologic study of 540 patients. Obstet Gynecol 56: 419–426

Blythe J G, Hodel K A, Wahl T P et al 1986 Para-aortic node biospy in cervical and endometrial cancers: does it affect survival? Obstet Gynecol 155: 306–314

Boronow R C 1969a Therapeutic considerations in endometrial cancer. J Miss State Med Assoc 10: 451–456

Boronow R C 1969b Carcinoma of the corpus: treatment at M. D. Anderson Hospital. In: Cancer of the Uterus and Ovary. Year Book, Chicago, pp 35–61

Boronow R C 1973 Editorial comment: a fresh look at corpus cancer management. Obstet Gynecol 42: 448–451

Boronow R C 1976 Endometrial cancere, not a benign disease. Obstet Gynecol 47: 630–634

Boronow R C 1980 Staging of endometrial cancer. Int J Radiat Oncol Biol Phys 6: 355–359

Boronow R C, Moderator 1987 Endometrial cancer work-shop. Unpublished material, International Gynecologic Cancer Society, Amsterdam

Boronow R C 1990 Advances in diagnosis, staging and management of cervical and endometrial cancer, stage I and II. Cancer 65: 648–659

Boronow R C 1991 Clinical opinion: should whole pelvic radiation therapy become past history? A case for the routine use of extended field therapy and multimodality therapy. Gynecol Oncol 43: 71–76

Boronow R C, Morrow C P, Creasman W T et al 1984 Surgical staging in endometrial cancer: clinical–pathologic findings of a prospective study. Obstet Gynecol 63: 825–832

Cheon H D 1969 Prognosis of endometrial carcinoma. Obstet Gynecol 34: 680–684

Creasman W T, Morrow C P, Bundy B N et al 1987 Surgical pathologic spread patterns of endometrial cancer: a gynecologic oncology group study. Cancer 60: 2035–2041

DiSaia P J, Creasman W T, Boronow R C et al 1985 Risk factors and recurrent patterns in stage I endometrial cancer. Obstet Gynecol 151: 1009–1015

Feuer G A, Calanog A 1987 Endometrial carcinoma: treatment of positive paraortic nodes. Gynecol Oncol 27: 104–109

Homesley H O, Boronow R C, Lewis J L Jr 1976 Treatment of adenocarcinoma of the endometrium at Memorial–James Ewing Hospitals, 1949–1965. Obstet Gynecol 47: 100–105

Inoue T, Morita K 1988 Five-year results of postoperative extended-field irradiation on 76 patients with nodal metastases from cervical carcinoma stage IB to IIIB. Cancer 61: 2009–2014

Kistner R W, Reagan J W, Krantz K E et al 1973 Endometrial cancer: rising incidence, detection and treatment. J Reprod Med 10: 53–74

Komaki R, Mattingly R F, Hoffman R G et al 1983 Irradiation of para-aortic lymph node metastases from carcinoma of the cervix or endometrium. Radiology 147: 245–248

Lewis B V, Stallworth J A, Cowdell R 1970 Adenocarcinoma of the body of the uterus. J Obstet Gynecol Br Commonw 77: 343–348

Morrow C P, DiSaia P F, Townsend D E 1973 Current management of endometrial carcinoma. Obstet Gynecol 42: 399–406

Morrow C P, Bundy B N, Kurman R J et al 1991 Relationship between surgical–pathological risk factors and outcome in clinical stage I and II carcinoma of the endometrium: a gynecologic oncology group study. Gynecol Oncol 40: 55–65

Pettersson F (ed) 1989 Annual report on the results of treatment in gynecological cancer, vol 20. International Federation of Gynecology and Obstetrics, Stockholm

Pettersson F (ed) 1991 Annual report on the results of treatment in gynecological cancer, vol 21. International Federation of Gynecology and Obstetrics, Stockholm

Plentl A A, Friedman E A 1971 Lymphatic system of the female genitalia. In: The morphologic basis of oncologic diagnosis and therapy. Saunders, Philadelphia

Potish R A, Twiggs L B, Adcock L L et al 1984 The utility and limitations of decision theory in the utilization of surgical staging and extended field radiotherapy in cervical cancer. Obstet Gynecol Surv 39: 555–562

Potish R A, Twiggs L B, Adcock L L et al 1985 Paraortic lymph node radiotherapy in cancer of the uterine corpus. Obstet Gynecol 65: 251–256

Rotman M, Moon S, John M et al 1978 Extended field para-aortic radiation in cervical carcinoma: the case for prophylactic treatment. Int J Radiat Oncol Biol Phys 4: 795–799

Rubin S C, Brookland R, Mikuta J J et al 1984 Para-aortic nodal metastases in early cervical carcinoma: long-term survival following extended-field radiotherapy. Gynecol Oncol 18: 213–217

Rutledge F 1974 The role of radical hysterectomy in adenocarcinoma of the endometrium. Gynecol Oncol 1: 331–347

Stallworthy J A 1971 Surgery of endometrial cancer in the Bonney tradition, Ann R Coll Surg Engl 48: 293–305

Webster's Ninth New Collegiate Dictionary 1989. Merriam–Webster, Springfield, MA.

13

Obstetric and gynaecological injuries of the urinary tract: their prevention and management

Richard Turner-Warwick   C. R. Chapple

The proximity of the female genital and the lower urinary tracts naturally results in a degree of structural and functional interdependence that make occasional urinary tract complications inevitable after childbirth and gynaecological procedures.

The traditional boundaries between some areas of surgical specialization are inappropriate to the proper development and improvement of our care of patients — this is reflected in the evolution of a number of regional surgical specialities, such as head and neck surgery, hand surgery, etc. Thus, within the traditional confines of gynaecology and urology, we have to recognize the need for cross-boundary training and sub-specialization by the development of specialist interests in uro-gynaecology and gynaeco-urology. The natural progress of this must be the development of a small number of referral units with a special experience in pelvic surgery for the treatment of complex congenital, traumatic, oncological and radiotherapeutic problems — the days of amateur 'committee surgery' in the pelvis must surely be numbered.

THE SURGICAL SIGNIFICANCE OF INFREQUENT VOIDING

A common urological complication of obstetric and gynaecological procedures is the development of voiding dysfunction—ranging from 'difficulty' to retention. It is fundamentally important to appreciate that this is usually the result of an exacerbation of a pre-existing extreme of normal function — infrequent voiding. Patients who void infrequently, sometimes at intervals of 4–6 hours or more, are prone to develop voiding difficulties after even minimal pelvic surgery and, incidentally, they are also prone to late-onset urinary infection (Turner-Warwick 1978, Turner-Warwick & Whiteside 1979, Turner-Warwick & Kirby 1991). The quick way to identify a patient's overall voiding pattern is to ask them one simple direct question: 'Is your usual voiding habit hourly, 2-hourly or 4-hourly?'. Simple subsidiary questioning of the 4-hour group then identifies the '6-hour-plus' and the occasional 'twice-a-day' patient, and this important urological fact should be included in every preoperative pelvic surgery history. Hourly voiding naturally raises the suspicion of a hypersensory or an unstable bladder.

211

However, the 'unexpected' complication of postoperative voiding inefficiency among infrequent voiders is by no means confined to a disturbance after local pelvic surgery; it can develop as an indirect complication of unrelated surgical procedures such as hip arthroplasty. Since the development of post-hysterectomy bladder-base descent is particularly likely to exacerbate a subclinical voiding inefficiency in patients who void infrequently, a simple elevating–repositioning of the vault closure with the round ligament is generally advisable to reduce the incidence (Turner-Warwick 1978).

The anxieties involved in repeated urethral re-catheterization after a trial of voiding — the so-called 'yo-yo catheter' — are best anticipated and obviated by routine postoperative suprapubic catheter drainage of infrequent voiders. A 16–18 F catheter should be used for this, because it takes an inconveniently long time to drain a post-voiding residual for monitoring measurement if smaller sizes are used.

It is especially important for gynaecological surgeons to recognize that, characteristically, patients who void infrequently usually have thin-walled bladders and that this predisposes them to the development of an ischaemic supratrigonal vesico-vaginal fistula after a simple hysterectomy (see below).

Patients who develop postoperative voiding difficulties after an operation are sometimes positively indignant about the situation because they regard their socially convenient infrequent voiding as 'excellent bladder function'. Having identified this situation from the preoperative history it is wise to forewarn them that their infrequent voiding can cause problems postoperatively. If such a patient should develop voiding difficulties or a fistula, such a forewarning may help them to understand that it was the peculiarities of their bladder that predisposed to it — not simply a surgical misadventure. Thus preoperative awareness of the potential problems of infrequent voiding may be helpful both to the patient and to the surgeon.

OBSTETRIC INJURIES TO THE URINARY TRACT

Indirect injuries

There is increasing awareness that apparently normal and uncomplicated vaginal deliveries can cause significant neuromuscular damage to the pelvic floor and the sphincter mechanisms, and that this can later result in the development of pelvic floor prolapse and incontinence.

It is also important to recognize that a slow delivery under prolonged epidural anaesthesia can result in the asensory bladder becoming grossly over-distended — for hours on end — and this can induce a serious, long-lasting, postpartum voiding dysfunction in patients whose previous bladder function was quite normal. Careful monitoring of the urinary output, at least 4-hourly and by catherization when necessary, is essential to avoid an occasionally severe bladder dysfunction in such patients.

Direct injuries

Direct fistulous injury to the urinary tract during a natural delivery is an unusual event in medically developed countries. However, worldwide, it is the commonest cause of urinary–vaginal fistulae. These fistulae result from prolonged obstructed labour in which the fetal head compresses the bladder base against the pubis, causing ischaemic pressure necrosis. When this involves circumferential damage to the proximal urethra it often results in disastrous sphincter destruction.

All procedures used to assist a marginally difficult vaginal delivery inevitably carry some risk of paravaginal injury that may involve the bladder base or urethra. Injuries associated with forceps delivery are naturally the commonest and the actual incidence of these generally reflects the experience and the judgement of the obstetrician. The bladder is particularly vulnerable in the course of a Caesarean delivery and, occasionally, one or even both ureters may be involved.

Rupture of the uterus resulting from a trial of labour after a previous Caesarean delivery tends to involve the bladder as a result of secondary adhesions between its posterior surface and the lower segment scar. The consequent vesical disruption can be extensive and may extend downwards into the urethra, causing severe injury to the sphincter mechanism.

The traditional and largely discontinued procedure of pubiotomy, in which the pubic symphysis is divided with a Gigli saw, can be a source of complications. The consequent pubic diastasis can, in itself, result in disruption of the anterior wall of the urethra due to the bilateral tethering of the lateral components of the pubo-urethral ligament that is divided in the midline. The misguided initial passage of the Gigli saw up the urethra itself naturally results in the predictable disaster of a coincidental full-length and full-thickness urethrotomy. The practice of delivery in the exaggerated lithotomy position can even result in a spontaneous pubic fracture–diastasis urethral injury if the hips are forcibly flexed.

Termination of pregnancy

Bladder injuries due to instrumental perforation of the uterus are a well-recognized complication of termination of a pregnancy, particularly in inexperienced hands. Among the more unusual is a perforating injury caused by the teeth of Volsellum forceps erroneously applied to a fold of the anterior vagina and the underlying bladder wall instead of the cervix.

THE CAUSES AND PREVENTION OF GYNAECOLOGICAL SURGICAL INJURIES TO THE URINARY TRACT

Both the ureter and the bladder are vulnerable during pelvic surgery for both benign and malignant conditions. Direct gynaecological surgical injuries result in fistulation into the vagina from the ureter, from the bladder or from the urethra, or a combination of these. An autonomic pelvic neuropathy may result from a radical hysterectomy and cause a lasting dysfunction of previously normal bladder behaviour. This is rarely a significant factor in voiding difficulties that develop in infrequent voiders after a simple hysterectomy in which the line of resection is as close as possible to the surface of the supracervical segment.

Ureteric injury

The ureters are most commonly damaged during the course of the dissection and ligation of the lateral pedicles containing the uterine and vaginal vessels. They may be divided, windowed, or included in the ligature. The management of ureteric injuries is considered separately below.

The aetiology of post-hysterectomy vesico-vaginal fistulae

A vesico-vaginal fistula that develops after hysterectomy is commonly large and located in the mid-line above the trigone. Usually these do not become apparent immediately: the vaginal leakage of urine usually starts a few days postoperatively. Such fistulae are commonly the result of a small area of ischaemia that develops following the separation of the natural adhesion of the posterior wall of a thin-walled bladder from its natural adhesion to the anterior surface of the uterus and cervix (Turner-Warwick 1993). These fistulae are not common but they are more likely to occur in patients who void infrequently, not only because their bladders are particularly thin walled, but also because they are prone to develop a postoperative voiding efficiency, and over-distension of the bladder predisposes to the development of ischaemic necrosis of the thin, detached and precariously vascularized supratrigonal area.

Even the most experienced gynaecological surgeons are not entirely immune from this fortuitous complication: it is best avoided by meticulously careful mobilization of the bladder, by scissor dissection rather than the traditional blunt 'push-off' separation with a dry swab, and especially by the avoidance of postoperative bladder distension by careful suprapubic catheter monitoring of the voiding efficiency postoperatively.

Anterior colporrhaphy

Injury to the urethra is a rare but well-recognized complication of anterior colporrhaphy, usually in association with a severe postoperative wound infection. The development of a urethro-vaginal fistula is particularly serious because of the associated damage to the intrinsic urethral sphincter mechanism. The particular problems associated with the repair of these are considered below.

Neo-vaginoplasty fistulae

Various surgical options are available for the creation of a neo-vaginal lining. Split-skin and amnion can be satisfactory substitutes but both have the disadvantage that the wall of the neo-vagina is not only very thin but its capacity is relatively small and tends to contract. Thus its size needs to be maintained by regular intercourse or by the passage of dilators and this can occasionally result in neo-vaginal rupture and the development of a fistula into the rectum or the bladder. The resolution of neo-vaginal fistulae presents particular problems and an omento-neo-vaginoplasty can be a useful retrieval procedure (Turner-Warwick 1986b,c, 1993). Caecolo-vaginoplasty (Turner-Warwick & Ashken 1967, Kirby & Turner-Warwick 1990) offers particular advantages, not only for the primary creation of a vagina but also for the resolution of neo-vaginal contraction and fistulae. The result is not only relatively robust but also it does not tend to contract, so that regular use or dilation is not required to maintain an adequate capacity. This is a particular advantage when neo-vaginoplasty is required early in puberty for haematometra.

Para-vaginal 'cysts'

Sequestrated elements of persistent congenital ducts tend to become cystic but, occasionally, their surgical excision can prove to be a trap for the unwary. An obstructed duplication of the upper urinary tract can masquerade as a para-vaginal cyst and a local excision naturally results in a uretero-vaginal fistula. The excision of 'cystic' urethral diverticula presents particular problems (see below) and the complications escalate in intersex variations, such as the adreno-genital syndrome, when the sphincter mechanisms have a somewhat male configuration.

THE AVOIDANCE OF SURGICAL INJURIES TO THE URINARY TRACT

The basic essential for the avoidance of any particular postoperative complication is to anticipate the possibility that it might arise.

Surgical access

The confines of the pelvic cavity present a natural restriction to surgical access — the less experienced the surgeon, the more important it is to obtain the best possible surgical exposure. A major and avoidable factor that predisposes to pelvic surgical complications is the additional restriction of surgical access created by the traditional combination of the classic Pfannensteil incision and a relatively inefficient retractor system, such as Balfour-type self-retaining instrument or those that are hand-held by assistants. Surgeons in general, and those in training in particular, could find that their routine pelvic surgical procedures are considerably simplified by the improved access provided by the simple 'suprapubic V' modification of the Pfannensteil incision with an efficient ring-retractor system.

The 'suprapubic V' incision

The 'suprapubic V' procedure uses a skin incision that is identical to that of a Pfannensteil procedure but it makes much better use of the local anatomy to provide a greatly improved surgical exposure — not only of the pelvis but also the lower abdomen (Fig. 13.1) (Turner-Warwick et al 1974, Turner-Warwick 1992, 1993).

It is a general-purpose incision for all lower abdominal and pelvic surgery, including a reflux–preventing reimplantation of the mid-ureter into the bladder, above the iliac vessels, using the BEPH procedure (see below). Thus, an unextended V incision provides good proximal access to the middle third of the ureter and it can be extended upwards and laterally into a supracostal incision for a synchronous nephrectomy. However, this proximal extension does not provide good access to the stomach, in the mid-line, for the mobilization of the omentum; consequently it is not appropriate for fistula repair (see below).

Abdominal access to the pelvis is also greatly increased by ring retraction. The universal Turner-Warwick perineo-abdominal ring-retractor, with its half-curved abdominal wall rectactor-retaining blades, maximizes the exposure provided by any incision (Fig. 13.2). The circumferential disposition of appropriately shaped deep-retraction blades and multiple traction stay-sutures, retained by the tips of haemostats tucked under the margin of the ring, elevates the bladder and the vaginal vault and eliminates the need to use an assistant as a retractor.

Surgical technique and tissue handling

Uncomplicated surgery is all about technique and tissue handling. Most surgeons regard their surgical technique as meticulous and immaculate. However, simple observation reveals that some surgeons and some instruments are more tissue sensitive than others. For instance, tissue forceps applied to structures that will remain in situ should be gentle enough to apply to a fold of one's finger skin without causing pain. Allis forceps are distinctly tissue crushing, and would-be reconstructive surgeons who use them might do well to take a course in micro-surgery in an endeavour to improve their concepts of technique and tissue handling.

Dexon and Vicryl sutures cause much less tissue reaction than catgut. Size for size they are much stronger and they retain their tensile strength longer, so that several sizes smaller can be used. The author thankfully abandoned catgut for all urinary tract operations in 1970 when Davis and Geck pioneered

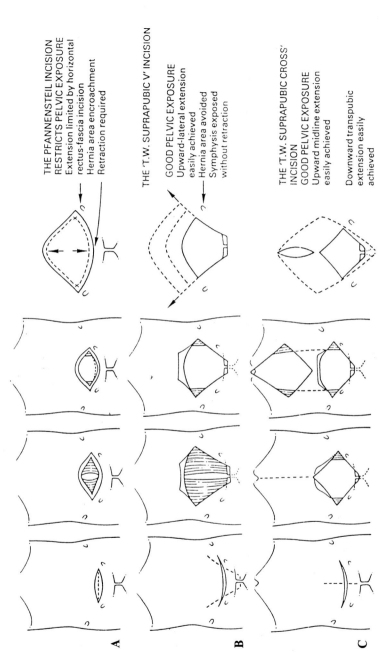

THE PFANNENSTEIL INCISION RESTRICTS PELVIC EXPOSURE
Extension limited by horizontal rectus-fascia incision
Hernia area encroachment
Retraction required

THE 'T.W. SUPRAPUBIC 'V' INCISION
GOOD PELVIC EXPOSURE
Upward-lateral extension easily achieved
Hernia area avoided
Symphysis exposed without retraction

THE 'T.W. SUPRAPUBIC CROSS' INCISION
GOOD PELVIC EXPOSURE
Upward midline extension easily achieved
Downward transpubic extension easily achieved

Fig.13.1. A The traditional Pfannensteil incision provides a relatively restricted surgical access to the pelvis. The lateral extent of its horizontal incision in the rectus sheath is limited by the inguinal canal area and the lower margin of the rectus sheath requires retraction. **B** The TW suprapubic V incision uses the same horizontal skin incision but the access of the pelvis and the lower abdomen is greatly improved. An initial 4 cm horizontal incision is made into the rectus sheath 2 cm *below* the upper margin of the pubis. Laterally, the incision in the rectus sheath is angled obliquely upwards so that the base width of the consequent 'V' flap does not extend beyond the lateral border of the rectus muscle, into the lateral abdominal muscles — unless a definitive upward extension is required. The distal extent of the incision provides a wide exposure of the upper border of the pubis and, because the distal margin of the rectus sheath is prepubic, it does not require retraction to provide full access to the retropubic space. **C** The 'TW suprapubic cross' incision also uses the same horizontal skin incision but its sub-umbilical mid-line incision in the abdominal wall can be extended upwards to provide supra-umbilical upper abdominal access for mobilization of the right gastro-epiploic pedicle of the omentum from the stomach by using an additional vertical epigastric mid-line skin incision. © 1974 Institute of Urology.

A

B

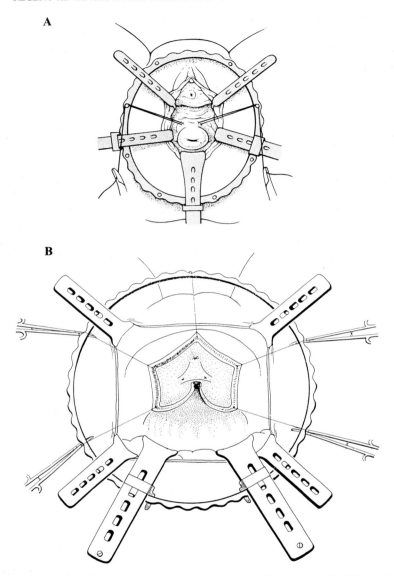

Fig.13.2.   The Turner-Warwick universal perineo-abdominal ring retractor. **A**   The perineal ring retractor has malleable copper vaginal blades. Traction stay sutures are used to pull a fistula area down to the introitus and guide knobs control their direction. **B**   The curved abdominal blades of the abdominal ring retractor retract the abdominal wall and hold the ring firmly in position. The deep blades have a retaining slide-hook that holds them in position. Traction stay sutures retained by haemostat tip under the ring margins elevate the bladder and vaginal vault for fistula repairs. No retractor hand-held by an assistant is required. © 1970 Institute of Urology.

the production of PGA sutures. Although PGA causes a relatively mild tissue reaction in the course of their dissolution it is easy to create an excessive tissue reaction by the mass ligation of a bulky pedicle that strangulates a large cuff of tissue.

THE PRINCIPLES OF REPAIR OF URINARY FISTULAE

Direct injuries to the urinary tract resulting from gynaecological surgery and from childbirth commonly result in fistulation into the vagina from the ureter, from the bladder or from the urethra, or a combination of these. Each of these three distinct fistulae presents a different surgical problem involving quite separate considerations; occasionally the rectum may also be involved.

It is almost invariably possible to close a urinary vaginal fistula. Meticulous technique is naturally essential, but reliable success with the more complicated problems is dependent upon the ability and inclination of the surgeon to select the procedure that is best suited to the particular clinical situation and, furthermore, to vary it according to the findings in the course of the operation on the basis of a wide personal experience.

The principles of layer closure of a fistula

The basic principles of the layer closure of a fistula are well established but there are many technical options.

After appropriate separation of the vagina and bladder, facilitated by a guiding finger in the vagina, the abnormal tissue at the margin of the fistula is resected. Modern surgeons usually use PGA sutures in preference to catgut, and knots are tied on the lumen whenever possible so that their bulk falls away without causing additional tissue reaction. If the tissue quality of the bladder is sufficiently good for a simple layer closure procedure it is simply closed with two layers of sutures. However, if there is any doubt whatsoever about the success of a simple layer closure procedure, an interposition support procedure is advisable.

Supporting the closure of complex fistulae by interposition grafts

When the healing potential of the tissue around a fistula is compromised by fibrotic scar tissue, resulting from infection, from the failure of previous repairs or from irradiation, the reliability of a simple layer closure procedure diminishes abruptly unless an additional well-vascularized transposition graft is interposed. The advisability of interposition support usually becomes obvious in the course of an operation so that, in general, surgeons should regard the recurrence of a fistula after a simple layer closure procedure as an avoidable complication even though it may be fortuitously inevitable on occasion.

The Martius labial-fat flap is a time-honoured procedure for the bulk support of a vaginal closure. However, fat is a relatively inert and poorly vascularized tissue. A sizeable flap of para-pelvic peritoneum sometimes provides sufficient additional interposition support for an abdominal layer closure but it is generally inappropriate when it is also involved in the local pathology — especially irradition. Pedicled muscle flaps, such as gracilis, can be used as a simple tissue-bulk interposition; however, skeletal muscle is ill-adapted to resist infection and to resolve inflammation so it can contribute little to the local healing reaction. Its vascular response potential is primarily exercise related and, ultimately, inactivity results in disuse atrophy and fibrosis. The omentum is the only body tissue that is specifically developed for the resolution of inflammation and healing so that, functionally, it is the ideal interposition tissue (see below).

THE TIMING OF REPAIR

Because urinary fistulae in the female are commonly the result of gynaecological and obstetric complications, in addition to the most unpleasant inconvenience for the patient, they often present a medicolegal aspect. The essential of treatment is to resolve the situation as early as possible without any complications — failure to achieve this should be a very rare event.

The major change in the management of postoperative vesical and ureteric fistulae in recent years has been proceeding to an immediate repair whenever possible, in preference to the traditional delayed repair that was advocated to ensure that the local tissue reaction had settled (Turner-Warwick 1993). Early diagnosis and immediate specialist referral are therefore important because, after 2 weeks, the local healing reaction tends to make a repair rather more difficult and precarious so it may then be advisable to defer it for 2–3 months or more. *Thus a gynaecological surgical fistulae should be regarded as a urological emergency.*

However, this generalization does not usually apply to *urethro-vaginal* fistulae because these are inherently associated with damage to the all-important intrinsic urethral sphincter mechanism upon which continence depends; the appropriate procedure for these is usually a delayed definitive reconstructive sphincteroplasty (see below). Similarly the postpartum tissue changes may make an immediate repair of some obstetric fistulae inadvisable.

Even relatively small vesico-vaginal fistulae rarely respond to conservative treatment by simple catheter drainage of the bladder; an immediate procedure with definitive closure is generaly advisable because 'hopeful delay' is likely to result in deferment of the repair for 2–3 months until the local reaction has settled. However, when the layer closures are separated by an omental interposition success is less dependent upon the local healing, so the timing is less critical. Thus the timing of a repair must be carefuly considered in relation to each particular case.

The collection of incontinent urine

When it is necessary to postpone the repair of a vaginal urinary fistula for a few months the collection of incontinent urine becomes a major problem in the unfortunate patient's life. However, the deferment should be carried through with fortitude until the appropriate time because disasters can lurk in inappropriate attempts at premature closure. Unfortunately, all too often there is no alternative to simple absorbent pads. Sometimes the urine leakage from a small vaginal fistula can be helpfully reduced by indwelling urethral catheter drainage but this is usually inefficient when the fistula is large. When the calibre of the vaginal introitus is narrow enough to retain a 40–50 ml catheter balloon, vaginal catheter drainage is an effective and under-used technique, for both vesico-vaginal and uretero-vaginal fistulae.

THE PRINCIPLES OF THE MANAGEMENT OF VESICO-VAGINAL FISTULAE

The closure of even an apparently simple vesico-vaginal fistula should be regarded as a specialist gynaeco-urological or uro-gynaecological procedure. The surgeon who creates a fistula is not usually the best person to undertake its repair. Postoperative fistulae are not common and an experience of the various options, based upon repairs of an individual surgeon's own fistulae complications, must be very limited. From the medicolegal point of view, apart from resolving a situation as early as possible, it is most important to ensure the uncomplicated success of the closure. An analysis of a personal series of some 300 fistula repairs over the years clearly shows that the difficulty tends to escalate when the situation becomes complex as the result of previous surgical failures or irradiation.

Preoperative evaluation

Careful preoperative evaluation and identification of a fistula is, of course, essential — not forgetting that there may be more than one. The standard procedures for this are well described. Urographic proof that the ureters are draining freely into the bladder and have not been involved in the vesical damage is particularly important. It is generally helpful and advisable to insert ureteric catheters into the ureters as an immediate preliminary to protect their orifices during a vesical repair and to facilitate their identification extravesically during an abdominal procedure, especially after a previous surgical failure or irradiation.

The repair approach options

The basic surgical option for the repair of a vesical fistula lies between a vaginal approach procedure and an abdominal approach procedure. Many surgeons have an instinctive personal preference for one or other of these but this is not as it should be.

Although many simple vesico-vaginal fistulae can be closed by a vaginal repair procedure the access that this provides is relatively restricted and almost any incidence of failure after this suggests under-usage of the abdominal approach. Similarly, a significant incidence of failure after a simple abdominal approach layer closure can be resolved by a formal omental interposition procedure, because in the absence of active tumour or infection this procedure should be almost invariably successful (Turner-Warwick et al 1967, Turner-Warwick 1976, 1986b,c).

The vaginal approach repair

A vaginal approach layer-closure is well described in standard texts. If there is any doubt about the quality of a simple layer-closure an additional Martius labial fat flap interposition procedure can be used.

Instrumentation

Appropriate instrumentation greatly facilitates the restricted access of vaginal surgery. The perineal element of the TW universal perineo-abdominal ring retractor system has malleable copper blades for vaginal retraction posteriorly and posterolaterally (Fig. 13.2): the guide knobs maintain the direction of traction stay sutures used to draw a fistula down towards the introitus and this greatly improves the surgical access — it is a more efficient retractor for reconstructive vaginal surgery than the traditional weighted Auvard instrument and it also obviates the necessity of a retracting surgical assistant — for whom there is relatively little room during the perineal component of a synchronous perineo-abdominal repair procedure (see below).

Two instruments have been specifically designed to facilitate restricted access surgery and are particularly valuable for vaginal surgery in general and complex fistula closure in particular (Fig. 13.3).

1. The TW needle holders are gently curved to keep the hand out of the 'line of sight' of the needle. This is particularly helpful for accurate suturing when surgical access to a delicate reconstruction deep in the pelvis or high in the vagina is unavoidably restricted.

2. The TW fibre-light sucker provides an invaluable combination of 'suck and see' in deep dark places. It is also appropriately curved.

The abdominal approach repair procedures

Even if a preoperative decision has been made to use an abdominal approach repair procedure a synchronous vaginal access is a great advantage; in particular a guiding finger in the vagina facilitates development of the plane of separation and haemostasis. This is provided by the PAPA perineo-abdominal progression approach (see below).

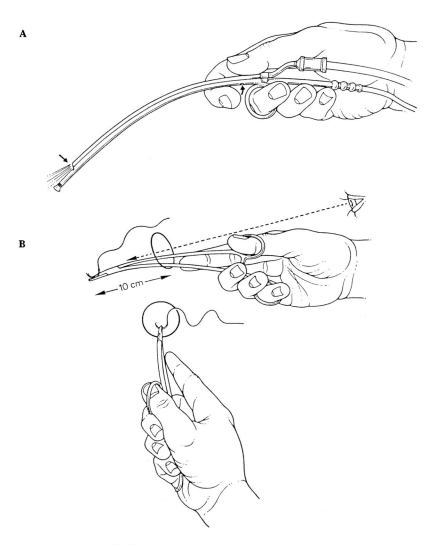

Fig.13.3 A The TW fibre-light sucker provides an invaluable combination of 'suck and see' in deep dark places. It is appropriately curved, with a suction hold at the distal end of the fibre-light to keep it blood free and a suction pressure-reducing hole in the trigger finger position beyond the middle finger ring-handle. **B** The TW needle holder is gently curved to keep the hand out of the line of sight of the needle. This is particularly helpful when surgical access to a delicate reconstruction is unavoidably restricted. © 1977 Institute of Urology.

The trans-peritoneal supravesical approach

The traditional anterior trans-vesical approach provides only a relatively restricted exposure for a simple layer closure of a fistula — it is no longer advocated and should be abandoned. The trans-peritoneal supravesical approach provides the best exposure for the repair of vesico-vaginal fistulae (Fig. 13.4). It facilitates separation of the vagina from the back of the bladder and the urethra. It enables the separation of the vagina to be extended into an effectively wide abdomino-perineal tunnel for omental interposition, should this be indicated (see below).

This approach facilitates a reflux-preventing reimplantation of the ureter when one or both of these are involved in the fistulous margin (see below). A synchronous perineo-abdominal urethral sphincteroplasty can be performed when a vesical fistula extends downwards through the bladder neck, creating an additional urethral defect (see below).

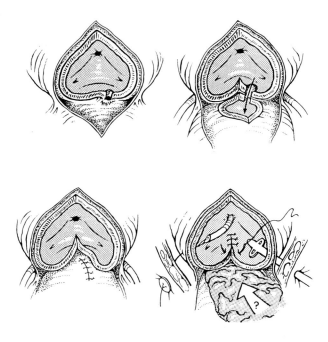

Fig.13.4 The supra-vesical approach for fistula repair. The posterior wall of the bladder and the vault of the vagina are exposed by appropriate deep ring retractor blades and elevating traction sutures. No retraction by an assistant is required. The bladder is opened down into the fistula by a laterally curved incision that facilitates closure. The vagina is separated from the bladder by scissor dissection, guided from below by a finger in the vagina. When appropriate, the separation of the vagina is extended down behind the urethra to the introitus to create an abdomino-perineal tunnel so that the mobilized omentum can be interposed between the layer closures of the bladder and vagina. © 1977 Institute of Urology.

It is most important that the incision in the posterior wall of the bladder should be laterally curved whenever the tissues are somewhat rigid as a result of irradiation or inflammatory fibrosis. This enables the bladder to be closed by an appropriate rotation of the consequently mobile and supple flap of the bladder wall. After irradiation a vertical mid-line incision in the bladder can prove impossible to close by simple side-to-side reapproximation.

The surgical value of omental redeployment support

Whenever there is any doubt about the quality of a simple adbominal approach layer closure an inter-position of pedicled omentum is indicated. Provided an adequate bulk of omentum is appropriately mobilized and interposed between PGA-sutured closure lines of the vagina and the bladder/urethra it can virtually guarantee the closure of even a complex vesico-vagino-rectal fistula (Fig. 13.5).

The omentum is unique in that it is the only body tissue that is specifically developed for the resolution of inflammation. This function is partly due to its vascularity, which is capable of rapid augmentation in response to inflammation; however, it is also fundamentally dependent upon its abundant lymphatic drainage, which is so good that it rapidly absorbs macro-molecular inflammatory exudates that can otherwise create purulent accumulations. Thus the omentum generally prevents abscess formation in the peritoneal cavity except in locations which it cannot reach, such as the pelvis and the sub-diaphragmatic areas (Turner-Warwick 1976).

Thus the omentum is invaluable for the support of the more precarious urinary tract reconstructions. Furthermore, because, unlike retroperitoneal and retropubic fat, the omentum always regains its suppleness after an inflammatory response has settled, it provides a unique urodynamic quality of support for functional reconstructions, such as vesicoplasty and sphincteroplasty, because it ensures the freedom of their functional expansion and movement (Turner-Warwick 1992a,b,c).

Mobilization of the omentum

The 'magic' of the omentum is dependent upon the 'pulsating efficiency' of its vascularization, and the preservation of this during its mobilization is essential to success. This is naturally dependent upon an accurate knowledge of its anatomical features.

The blood supply of the omentum is derived from the right gastro-epiploic branches of the gastroduodenal vessels and the left gastro-epiploic branches of the splenic vessels (Fig. 13.6). The right gastro-epiploic vascular pedicle is always larger than that of the left and there are only minor distal collateral anastomoses between the vertical branches of the gastro-epiploic arcade within the omental apron.

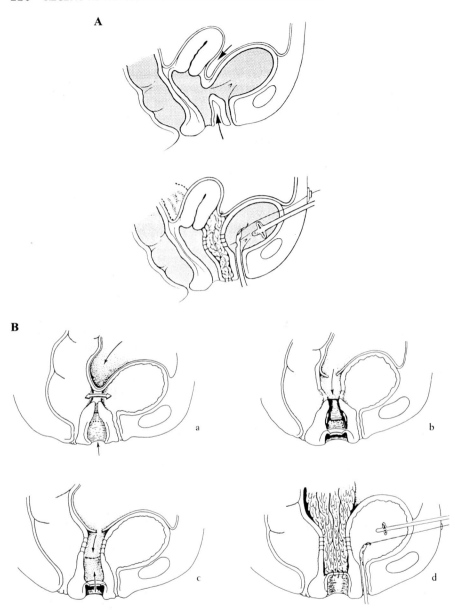

Fig.13.5. **A** Omental interposition for a recurrent vesico-vaginal fistula after the creation of a wide interposition abdomino-perineal tunnel. **B** The closure of a complex hysterectomy plus irradiation vesico-vaginal fistula achieved by excising the stenotic vault of the irradiated vagina to create a wide abdomino-perineal tunnel for omental interpositioning. © 1966 Institute of Urology.

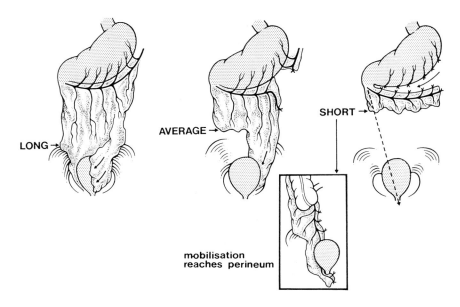

Fig.13.6. In 30% of cases the omental apron is long enough to reach the perineum after its simple separation from the transverse colon and meso-colon. In another 30% an additional division of its smaller left gastro-epiploic pedicle is required. Formal mobilization of the whole length of its right gastro-epiploic pedicle from the stomach is required in 40% — in such cases the pedicle should be protected by positioning it behind the mobilized right colon, and a prophylatic appendicectomy is generally advisable. © 1987 Institute of Urology.

In about 30% of patients the omentum will reach the perineum without definitive mobilization of its vascular pedicles. However, when it is surgically redeployed to support reconstructive procedures in the pelvis, it is generally advisable to separate its natural adhesion to the transverse colon and the mesocolon to avoid its distraction by postoperative gaseous distension of the bowel.

Simple division of its relatively minor left gastro-epiploic vascular pedicle enables a further 30% of omental aprons to reach the perineum and this does not significantly reduce its blood supply.

Thus, in about 40% of patients (more in children) meticulous full-length mobilization of the gastro-epiploic vascular pedicle from the stomach is required to enable it to be effectively redeployed in the pelvis. Because such a mobilized omentum is based on its narrow vascular pedicle it is anatomically advisable to protect this by mobilizing the right colon so that it can lie retroperitonally (Fig. 13.7).

Thus even when its apron is under-developed, as it often is in children, a normal omentum can always be redeployed into the pelvis. Unfortunately some surgical and gynaecological texts advocate basing the mobilization of the omentum upon its relatively minor vascular pedicle on the left; others even elongate the apron by a simple horizontal incision that transects its vertical vessels and this inevitably reduces its 'pulsating efficiency'. Furthermore, in about 10% of patients, there is no anastomotic junction between the right and the left gastro-epiploic vessels that usually form a complete gastro-epiploic arcade along the greater curvature of the stomach. The technical details of the mobilization of the omentum are detailed elsewhere (Turner-Warwick 1986a, b,c, 1992a,b, 1993).

In practice, an omental pedicle graft repair of a fistula in the pelvis is so reliable that complications and failures are almost always attributable to one or more of three shortcomings of surgical technique: (a) failure to develop an abdomino-perineal interposition tunnel of sufficient dimensions; (b) failure to mobilize an adequate bulk of omentum to fill the interposition tunnel; (c) impairment of the omental blood supply by an inappropriate vascular mobilization procedure (Fig. 13.7).

The 'three-option progression approach' procedure for vesico-urethro-vaginal fistulae

It is virtually always possible to close a vesico-vaginal fistula by the TOPA ('three-option (vaginal–abdominal–omental) progression approach') procedure, the details of which are described elsewhere (Turner-Warwick 1976,

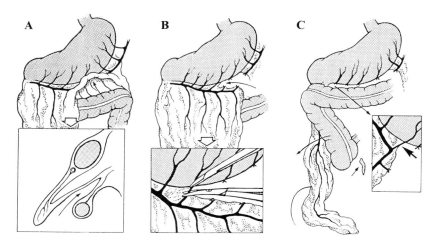

Fig.13.7. Mobilization of the right gastro-epiploic pedicle of the omentum requires meticulous vascular technique. **A** Separation from the transverse meso-colon by development of the avascular plane is always advisable to prevent postoperative displacement of the redeployed omentum by gaseous bowel distension. **B** Ligation in continuity reduces the risk of developing an interstitial haematoma. Ligation between the haemostats risks vessel escape; non-absorbable ligature material should always be used. **C** Once started, mobilization of the right gastro-epiploic vessels from the stomach should be extended to their gastroduodenal origin, otherwise tension on the pedicle at the point of the last undivided branch may rupture it. © 1977 Institute of Urology.

1986b,c, 1993). Almost the only indication for urinary diversion after a fistula operation is urinary incontinence due to irreparable sphincter damage.

The progression options are fundamental because, in reconstructive surgery, however detailed the preoperative evaluation, it is generally inappropriate to endeavour to decide, preoperatively, exactly how one will resolve a situation — especially when it is complex as a result of trauma, or persistent after previous surgical endeavours. The procedure should properly depend upon the findings at the time of surgery, and it can be most appropriately described (and, perhaps, most accurately scheduled preoperatively) as a 'TITBAPIT' (take it to bits and put it together) procedure' (Turner-Warwick 1986c, 1993).

Postoperative urine drainage

Double catheter is drainage an insurance against early postoperative bladder distension that can occasionally arise as a result of obstruction of the suprapubic catheter drainage. However, the use of a Foley balloon catheter is most inadvisable because inadvertent traction on this can disastrously disrupt a bladder base closure; a urethral catheter is best retained by a sling suture, button-fixed on the abdominal surface (see Fig. 13.5).

The PAPA (perineo-abdominal progression approach) operating position

The traditional 'exaggerated lithotomy' operating position that is generally used for vaginal-approach fistula repairs has serious shortcomings because it does not provide the facility of extension to a synchronous abdominal procedure in the event of necessity. The PAPA position is advocated for all intended vaginal-approach repairs because it combines adequate exposure, and facilitates the option of an extension to a synchronous perineo-abdominal procedure with minimal rearrangement.

The PAPA operating position (Fig. 13.8) enables the surgeon to move from one approach to the other, and back, during the operation, and a synchronous abdomino-perineal approach is, of course, essential for the proper development and distal perineal closure of the abdomino-perineal tunnel required for the omental interposition repair procedure.

During a definitive abdominal approach the synchronous vaginal access provided by the single sterile perineo-abdominal operating field of the PAPA position has many advantages: (a) it enables a finger in the vagina to guide the separation of the fused tissue layers around the fistula; (b) any bleeding that develops during the lateral development of an abdomino-perineal interposition tunnel can be immediately controlled by vaginal finger pressure until definitive haemostasis is secured; (c) it facilitates urethral catherization and manipulation; (d) endoscopic examination and instrumentation are occasionally helpful in the course of an operation.

However, in practice, the PAPA operating position is so convenient for the surgeon, for the scrub nurse and for the instrumentation that the author invariably uses it for all major abdomino-pelvic surgery — even when there is no expectation of need for a synchronous perineal approach or even a pelvic exploration.

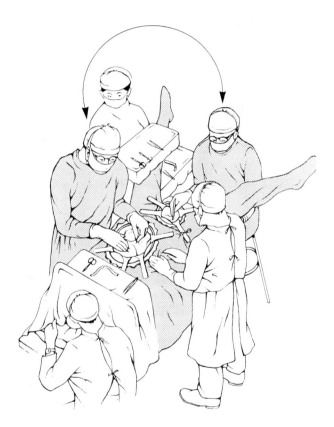

Fig.13.8.   The perineo-abdominal progression approach (PAPA) operating position for complex pelvic surgery. The patient is placed on the operating table in a flat, slightly head-down position and the legs are widely abducted with only moderate hip flexion. The perineum and abdomen are prepared and draped in a single sterile operating field. For a vaginal approach procedure, the surgeon is seated with the instrument table and scrub nurse immediately on the right (or left if left-handed). The bundle of suction tubing, fibre-light and diathermy cables is arranged over the patient's leg on the opposite side. When appropriate the surgeon simply walks round to the abdominal approach position and the scrub nurse repositions the instrument table between the patient's legs. It is rarely necessary to have two surgeons for a synchronous approach because the perineo-abdominal interchange is so simple. Furthermore, if appropriate ring retraction is used (both perineal and abdominal) one assistant is more than enough; certainly no assistant should intervene between the surgeon and the instrument table/scrub nurse. © 1977 Institute of Urology.

SOME COMPLEXITIES OF COMPLEX VESICO-VAGINAL FISTULAE

A fistula may be 'complex' as a result of impaired local tissue healing due to infection, to previous surgery or to irradiation. It may also be complicated by a congenital vaginal abnormality, by the additional involvement of the terminal ureter on one or both sides, by a urethral sphincter deficiency, by a coincident rectal fistula, or by a 'frozen pelvis' due to extensive radiation fibrosis. These complications naturally make a repair procedure more difficult but they are usually synchronously remediable by an appropriate variation of the available perineo-abdominal procedures.

The post-irradiation 'frozen pelvis'

Inevitably, the effective treatment of carcinoma of the cervix by radiotherapy results in a degree of irradiation tissue damage to the bladder and to the rectum. The extent of irradiation damage is not always directly related to the dose; there is considerable variation in the particular tissue response of the individual. Thus, a given depth dose that causes a moderate reaction in one patient may cause severe radiation fibrosis in another; sometimes this is sufficient to result in incarceration of the rectum and ureters — the so-called 'frozen pelvis' — and the development of a vesico-vaginal fistula which may be associated with a radio-necrotic cavity in the vaginal vault area.

Traditionally, such a 'frozen pelvis' used to be treated by a double abdominal surface urostomy and colostomy, but even this does not always relieve the unfortunate patient of an offensive purulent discharge from a radio-necrotic cavity. Although the fibrotic reaction in such cases is extensive, the anal canal, its sphincter mechanism and the lower segment of the vagina are rarely severely damaged (Fig. 13.9). Consequently it is often possible to exenterate the radiation fibrosis and to restore bowel continuity by anastomosis of the mobilized un-irradiated descending colon to the partially irradiated anal canal (Turner-Warwick 1986b, 1993). Such an anastomosis is potentially precarious but, provided it is meticulously performed, wrapped in a well-vascularized omental flap and protected by a loop-ileostomy, it is commonly successful.

The functional result of reconstructing a small-capacity irradiated bladder by a bowel substitution cystoplasty is primarily dependent upon whether the residual urethral sphincter mechanism is capable of maintaining continence. A cystoplasty/bladder-base anastomosis is also potentially precarious but, again, this is generally successful if a good omental support can be achieved. The anastomosis of the un-irradiated proximal ureter to the relatively un-irradiated bowel cystoplasty rarely presents difficulties.

The main additional problem involving the exenteration of a large mass of radiation fibrosis is the obliteration of the consequently large 'dead-space' cavity in the pelvis. Sometimes, redeployment of the whole of the omental

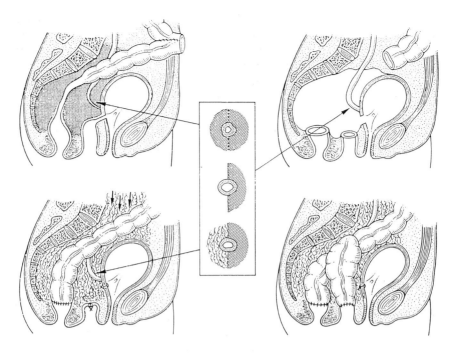

Fig. 13.9 Extensive resection/exenteration of the radiation fibrosis of a 'frozen pelvis' caused by the treatment of carcinoma of the cervix results in a rigid-walled cavity. Restoration of bowel continuity by colo-anal anastomosis is usually possible, and 'hemi-liberation' of obstructive ureteral incasement avoids the risk of necrosis resulting from circumferential mobilization. The pelvic 'dead-space' is best filled by redeployment of mobilized omentum when sufficient is available; otherwise the caecum can be used as a space-occupying structure. © 1975 Institute of Urology.

apron, on the basis of a full-length mobilization of its right gastro-epiploic vascular pedicle from the greater curvature of the stomach (Fig. 13.9), provides a sufficient bulk to fill this cavity. However, these patients are often somewhat emaciated so that even the fully mobilized omental apron is only sufficient to provide the critical vascular support for the actual suture line.

In such cases, the well-vascularized inverted colocaecal segment of the large bowel provides a satisfactory 'space-filling vaginoplasty' that effectively relines the margins of the exenteration cavity, the irradiation ischaemia of which prevents natural healing by proliferation of vascular granulation tissue (Turner-Warwick 1986b, 1993). The mucosal lining of such a 'neo-vaginal colo-cavity' naturally produces some mucous discharge but this is minimal, inoffensive and easily controllable (Kirby & Turner-Warwick 1990).

There is always a possibility of residual tumour cells in the fibrosis associated with an irradiation fistula, even when preoperative biopsies prove negative and even if the treatment was concluded 10 years or more previously. It is clearly inappropriate to attempt to close a fistula when the bulk of the pelvic induration associated with it is active, recurrent macroscopic tumour. However, when a patient develops a post-irradiation vesico-vaginal fistula and a representative preliminary biopsy shows only a few residual cells in extensive irradiation fibrosis, the local tumour may be relatively quiescent. Under these circumstances, because the prognosis is very poor, it is all the more important to resolve the incapacitating incontinence as swiftly and as efficiently as possible. Closure of such a fistula by omental interposition is not only a simpler procedure than a uretero-ileal surface conduit but it offers the patient a good chance of normal voiding and urinary control for their few short remaining months.

Urethral diverticulectomy and sphincter deficiency

Urethral diverticula are congenital out-pouchings of the urethral lining through its wall. They are commonly single and the neck of the diverticulum is usually located posteriorly about the junction of the proximal and middle third of the urethra. Becauses the whole 3–4 mm thickess of the urethral wall is formed by the all-important urethral sphincter muscles, all urethral diverticula are associatd with some degree of congenital sphincter deficiency and, consequently, a localized sphincter weakness.

Unfortunately, the sphincter deficiency associated with diverticula is commonly overlooked in their surgical treatment. Fistulation and urinary incontinence are not uncommon complications of simple diverticulectomy. The definitive excision of a urethral diverticulum should involve a definite reconstructive sphincteroplasty (Turner-Warwick 1993, Turner-Warwick & Kirby 1991, 1993).

Reconstructive urethral sphincteroplasty

The principle of reduction sphincteroplasty is to redeploy the remnants of the urethral sphincter to approximate to the normal anatomical distribution, with a synchronous reconstruction of the bladder neck mechanism. When appropriate the calibre of the urethral lumen is reduced to as little as 10–12 F to obtain a maximum bulk of sphincter approximation behind it (Fig. 13.10). This procedure was developed to restore the functional competence of the female urethra after traumatic injuries, the repair of urethro-vaginal fistula, the failure of simple urethral repositioning procedures for stress incontinence and for congenital deficiencies (Turner Warwick 1986a, 1992a,b,c, Turner-Warwick & Kirby 1992).

The functional success of a sphincteroplasty is additionally dependent upon the prevention of secondary peri-urethral fibrosis, which can immobilize its functional mobility by peripheral tethering; in complex situations this is best achieved by an omental interposition support, the urodynamic value of which is often under-appreciated.

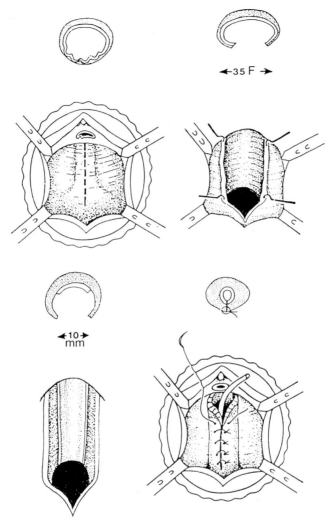

Fig.13.10. Reduction sphincteroplasty. The urethra is exposed through a hemi-circumferential introital pre-vaginal approach. The whole length of the urethra is opened posteriorly in the mid-line and the incision extended upwards, through the bladder neck into the trigone. A synchronous transvesical approach is required for a trigonal reduction/reconstruction of the calibre of the bladder neck mechanism because it is almost impossible to reduce accurately and reconstruct the trigone and bladder neck mechanism from below. Unnecessary mobilization of the lateral peri-urethral tissue is avoided because the innervation of the striated element of urethral sphincter mechanism is embedded in this. The 3 cm width of the opened urethral uro-epithelial lining is reduced to a 1 cm anterior strip and the urethral sphincter mechanism is overclosed around a 10 F stenting catheter, suture-slung through the abdominal wall. The functional success of a sphincteroplasty is additionally and essentially dependent upon the prevention of secondary peri-urethral fibrosis, which can immobilize its functional mobility by peripheral tethering. This is achieved by an omental interposition support, the urodynamic value of which is often under-appreciated. © 1982 Institute of Urology.

Sphincteroplasty is a surgically challenging procedure; each case presents its own peculiarities and, naturally, an anatomically satisfactory reconstruction of the residual sphincter mechanism does not necessarily create a satisfactory functional result.

Urethro-vaginal fistulae

The essential factor to bear in mind in the resolution of urethro-vaginal fistulae is that urinary incontinence is entirely dependent upon the function of the intrinsic urethral sphincter musculature within the thickness of the wall of the urethra.

If a bladder base injury extends down into the urethra to form a vesico-urethro-vaginal fistula it is invariably associated with a traumatic defect in the posterior sector of the urethral sphincter mechanism — just as a urethral diverticulum is associated with a congenital mid-posterior sector defect. Naturally, therefore, the appropriate procedure for the resolution of such a fistula is the extension of the vesical fistula repair to include a definitive repair of the sphincter (Fig. 13.10). This involves a synchronous combination of a perineal pre-vaginal reduction sphincteroplasty with an abdominal trans-vesical reconstruction of the bladder neck and mobilization of an omental support to ensure that its functional occlusive movement is not subsequently impaired by secondary peri-urethral fibrotic tethering (Turner-Warwick 1986a, 1992a,c). Without such a definitive extension of the reconstruction procedure, the risk of impaired urinary control is considerable.

The management of operative injury to the ureter and uretero-vaginal fistulae

Gynaecological surgical injuries to the ureter are generally located in its lower third. However, not infrequently, an associated ureteric injury is terminal, in conjunction with a vesical fistula; this emphasizes the importance of appropriate preoperative assessment of the upper urinary tracts.

The prevention of ureteric injury

A real awareness of the possibility that the ureter may be injured in the course of the pelvic surgery is the prime factor in its prevention. An accurate knowledge of the anatomy of the ureter — and, in particular, of its relationship to the vascular pedicle of the uterus and the ovary and also to the cervix — is essential. Good exposure is of paramount importance (see Fig. 13.1).

When there is any question of a complicated dissection due to uterine bulk, or to para-ureteric induration, infection or tumour, preliminary dissection–identification of the ureter is a wise precaution, assisted by the retrograde passage of a ureteric catheter or a 'fibre-light ureteric demonstrator'.

The timing of a definitive ureteric repair

Peroperative repair.   When a ureteric injury is identified at the time of surgery, and if it is not associated with a significant deficiency in its length, it is often possible to achieve a satisfactory restoration of continuity by an immediate spatulated overlap anastomotic repair. However, the delicacy of this procedure should not be underestimated, and its reliable success is certainly dependent upon meticulous reconstructive technique.

Early repair

A ureteric injury during hysterectomy commonly results in a vaginal leakage of urine that is apparent immediately postoperatively. The site of the leakage is usually revealed by an intravenous urogram because, almost always, the upper urinary tract is distended down to the level of the injury.

When a ureteric injury does not involve complete loss of ureteric continuity it is sometimes possible to circumnavigate it by the retrograde passage of a ureteric catheter. In such a case a double-J stent, left in-dwelling for 6–8 weeks, may be sufficient to resolve the situation. Otherwise a definitive surgical resolution is required.

Traditionally the repair of a ureteric injury has generally been a delayed procedure, but an immediate repair is currently advocated whenever possible. However, percutaneous nephrostomy has certainly simplified the immediate control of ureteric injury and initial management of upper urinary tract obstruction.

After the first few postoperative days the local peri-ureteric tissue reaction may compromise a simple end-to-end anastomic repair, especially when the lesion is low in the pelvis; however, the bladder elongation psoas-hitch (BEPH) procedure enables a lower-segment ureteric injury to be repaired at almost any time postoperatively. The great advantage of the resolution of a uretero-vaginal fistula by a uretero-neo-cystostomy is that the local inflammatory response associated with the injury is remote from, and does not involve, either the mid-ureter or the bladder at the site of the reimplantation. Consequently, the BEPH procedure can be used at any time postoperatively, provided no active acute inflammation is present.

The BEPH procedure

The myo-elastic properties of a normal bladder enable it to void to completion after a definitive elongation that enables it to reach above the iliac vessels, with suture anchoring to the psoas muscle for the reimplantation of the ureter. An important feature of this procedure is the initial, bladder-elongating hemi-circumferential incision into the 'equatorial line' of the bladder, because it is this that enables the dome of the bladder to be extended upwards, without tension, by at least the length of the hemi-circumferential incision of the bladder (Fig. 13.11) (Turner-Warwick & Worth 1969, Turner-Warwick 1988).

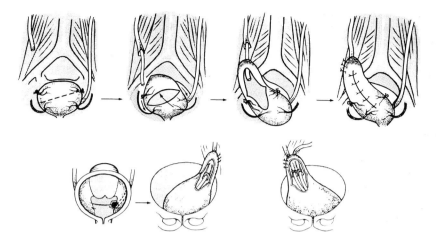

Fig.13.11.   The BEPH bladder elongation psoas-hitch procedure for replacement of the lower ureter. The overriding advantage of the BEPH procedure over the traditional Boari flap is that the relatively simple bladder elongation procedure achieved by the vertical closure of a horizontal hemi-circumferential incision in the equator of the bladder facilitates a reflux, preventing reimplantation of the normal middle third of the ureter into the normal relocated fundus of the bladder–well away from the local healing reaction at the side of the original ureteral injury in the pelvis. A single BEPH procedure can also be used for reimplantation of both ureters. © 1972 Institute of Urology.

The BEPH procedure has distinct advantages over the traditional Boari flap, because (a) the bladder incision is less than half the length; (b) the vascularization of the bladder extension is preserved (which is particularly important if the viability of the bladder wall is impaired by inflammation or irradiation); (c) a reflux-preventing tunnel reimplanation of the ureter into the elongated dome of the bladder is much easier than into a relatively narrow Boari flap; and bladder closure is greatly simplified.

When the lesion involves the lower part of the middle third of the ureter, or the bladder capacity is somewhat small, the extent of the bladder elongation can be increased by a strategic double incision (Turner-Warwick 1988, 1992a).

CONCLUSION

The traditional boundaries between some areas of surgical specialization are inappropriate to the proper development and improvement of our care of patients. This is reflected in the evolution of a number of regional surgical specialities, such as head and neck surgery, hand surgery, etc. Thus, within the traditional confines of gynaecology and urology, we have to recognize the need for cross-boundary training and specialization by the development of specialist interests in uro-gynaecology and gynaeco-urology. The natural progress of this must be the development of a small number of referral units with a special experience in pelvic surgery for the treatment of complex congenital, traumatic, oncological and radiotherapy problems. The days of amateur 'committee surgery' in the pelvis must surely be numbered.

Finally it is essential to appreciate that any operative procedure that fails, however well intentioned and however well performed, inevitably complicates a subsequent retrievoplasty — 'having a go' cannot be in the best interests of one's patients.

REFERENCES

Kirby R S, Turner-Warwick R 1990 Reconstruction of the vagina by caecolo-vaginoplasty. Surg Gynecol Obstet 170: 132–136
Turner-Warwick R 1976 The use of the omental pedicle graft in urinary tract reconstruction. J Urol 116: 341–347
Turner-Warwick R 1978 Impaired voiding efficiency and retention in the female. Clin Obstet Gynaecol 5: 193–207
Turner-Warwick R 1986a Female sphincter mechanisms and their relation to incontinence. In: Dubruyne F M J, Van Karrenbrock P E U A (eds) Surgery. Martinus Nijhof, Amsterdam, pp 66–75
Turner-Warwick R 1986b Vesico-vaginal fistula: the resolution of the 'frozen pelvis' by caeco vaginoplasty. In: Robb C, Smith R (eds) Operative surgery. Butterworth, London
Turner-Warwick R 1986c Urinary fistula in the female. In: Walsh P C et al (eds) Campbell's urology. Saunders, Philadelphia, pp 2718–2738
Turner-Warwick R 1988 The Turner-Warwick bladder elongation psoas hitch BEPH procedure for substitution ureteroplasty. In: Abrams, P, Gingell J C (eds) Controversies and innovations in urological surgery. Springer-Verlag, Berlin, Ch 39
Turner-Warwick R 1992a The anatomical basis of functional reconstruction of the urethra. In: Droller M (ed) Surgical anatomy. Mosby–Year Book, St Louis, Ch 61
Turner-Warwick R 1992b The functional anatomy of the urethra and its relation to the pelvic floor musculature. In: Mosby–Year Book, Droller M (ed) Surgical antomy. St Louis, Ch 60.
Turner-Warwick R 1992c Functional restoration of the incontinent female urethra. Rev Med Suisse Romande 112: 775–793
Turner-Warwick R 1993 The abdominal approach repair of vesico-vaginal fistulae. In: Nichols D (ed) Gynecologic and obstetric surgery. Mosby–Year Book, Philadelphia, Ch 53
Turner-Warwick R, Kirby R S 1991 Urodynamic studies and their effect upon management. In: Chisholm G D, Fair W R (eds) Scientific foundations of urology, 3rd edn. Heinemann, Oxford
Turner-Warwick R, Kirby R S 1993 Sphincteroplasty. In: Webster G et al (eds) Reconstructive urology. Blackwell Scientific Oxford, pp 657–686
Turner-Warwick R, Whiteside C G 1979 Clinical urodynamic. Urol Clin North Am 6: 13–30, 51–54, 259–264
Turner-Warwick R, Worth P H L 1969 The psoas-hitch procedure for the replacement of the lower third of the urethra. Br J Urol 41: 701–709
Turner-Warwick R, Worth P H L, Milroy E J G, Duckett J 1974 The 'supra-pubic V' incision. Br J Urol 46: 39–45.
Turner-Warwick R, Wynne E J C, Handley Ashken M 1967 The use of the omentum in the repair and reconstruction of the urinary tract. Br J Surg 54: 849

The Turner-Warwick range of instruments is supplied by V. Mueller, Chicago, by Leibinger, Germany, and by Downs and by Thackray, UK.

Index